101 Tips
for Behavior Change
in Diabetes
Education

Robert M. Anderson, EdD
Martha Mitchell Funnell, MS, RN, CDE
Nugget Burkhart, RN, MA, CPNP, CDE
Mary Lou Gillard, MS, RN, CDE
Robin Nwankwo, MPH, RD, CDE

American Diabetes Association.
Cure • Care • Commitment™

Director, Book Publishing, John Fedor; *Associate Director, Professional Books,* Christine B. Welch; *Editor,* Joyce Raynor; *Production Manager,* Peggy M. Rote; *Composition,* Circle Graphics, Inc.; *Cover Design,* Koncept Advertising and Design; *Printer,* Port City Press

Printed in the United States of America
1 3 5 7 9 10 8 6 4 2

The suggestions and information contained in this publication are generally consistent with the *Clinical Practice Recommendations* and other policies of the American Diabetes Association, but they do not represent the policy or position of the Association or any of its boards or committees. Reasonable steps have been taken to ensure the accuracy of the information presented. However, the American Diabetes Association cannot ensure the safety or efficacy of any product or service described in this publication. Individuals are advised to consult a physician or other appropriate health care professional before undertaking any diet or exercise program or taking any medication referred to in this publication. Professionals must use and apply their own professional judgment, experience, and training and should not rely solely on the information contained in this publication before prescribing any diet, exercise, or medication. The American Diabetes Association—its officers, directors, employees, volunteers, and members—assumes no responsibility or liability for personal or other injury, loss, or damage that may result from the suggestions or information in this publication.

⊗ The paper in this publication meets the requirements of the ANSI Standard Z39.48-1992 (permanence of paper).

ADA titles may be purchased for business or promotional use or for special sales. To purchase this book in large quantities, or for custom editions of this book with your logo, contact Lee Romano Sequeira, Special Sales & Promotions, at the address below, or at LRomano@diabetes.org or call 703-299-2046.

American Diabetes Association
1701 North Beauregard Street
Alexandria, Virginia 22311

Library of Congress Cataloging-in-Publication Data

101 tips for behavior change in diabetes education / Robert M. Anderson . . . [et al.].
    p. cm.
  ISBN 1-58040-149-X (pbk. : alk. paper)
    1. Diabetes—Psychological aspects—Miscellanea. 2. Patient education—Miscellanea. I. Title: One hundred one tips for behavior change in diabetes education. II. Anderson, Bob, EdD.

RC660.4 .A145 2002
616.4′62′019—dc21

                                                          2002027689

*To diabetes educators everywhere
who are dedicated
to improving the lives
of their patients.*

CONTENTS

Introduction vii

Approaches to Behavior Change 1

Assessment 11

Dealing with Emotion 17

Choosing to Change 23

Motivation 29

Attitudes, Beliefs, and Values 41

Goal-Setting 49

Social Support 61

Challenging Patients 69

Eating and Physical Activity 83

Educator–Patient Relationships 95

Help from Other Health Professionals 107

Educator Concerns 113

Pediatrics 125

INTRODUCTION

This book contains a series of tips for facilitating self-directed behavior change with people who have diabetes. Tips are included for helping patients across their life span who are facing a wide array of psychosocial and behavior-change challenges. The information in these tips reflect the philosophy, experiences, and practice of the diabetes educators at the University of Michigan Diabetes Research and Training Center. It is our hope that you will find these tips helpful in your practice.

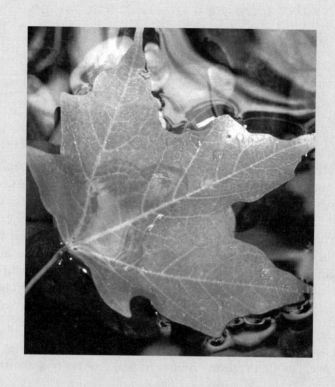

APPROACHES

TO BEHAVIOR

CHANGE

1

I know that there are a variety of theories for understanding and influencing health behavior. How can I decide which theory to use with my patients?

 Tip

There are two key principles to use when selecting a theory about behavior change. We'll call the first "experiential validity." As you read about a theory, you should ask yourself if it resonates with your own experience. In other words, does it seem consistent with the dynamics of behavior changes that you have made in your life and those that you have observed in the lives of others? No matter how much data exist to support the efficacy of a particular theoretical approach to behavior change, if the approach doesn't resonate with your experience, it is probably not a good choice for you.

The second principle is educational utility. Although a behavior-change approach needs to fit well with your experience, a good fit is not enough. The approach or theory must help you make decisions about how to work with patients in all settings. For example, if you were to choose the health belief model, you would probably help patients think about their perceived susceptibility to the complications of diabetes and the efficacy of the various self-management approaches in reducing their risk for those complications. If you were to choose the stages of change approach, you would assess your patients' stage of change relative to any particular diabetes self-management behavior.

2

I hear other educators talking about using patient empowerment as their philosophy of education. What does this mean?

 Tip

Almost all of the tips in this book reflect an underlying empowerment philosophy. At its most basic level, the empowerment philosophy means that as health care professionals, we realize that the responsibility for diabetes self-management rests with our patients. Furthermore, we realize that self-management is inseparable from the rest of the patient's life. The routine decisions patients make each day regarding nutrition, physical activity, and stress have a significant impact on their health and well-being. Our job is not to get patients to do what we consider "the right thing." Our responsibility is to help patients make informed decisions about diabetes and its self-management. Also, by engaging our patients in a nonjudgmental review of their current diabetes self-management, we can provide them with the opportunity to think about whether the decisions they are making are truly supporting their priorities and goals in life. Using an empowerment approach requires us to give up the notion that we can be responsible for our patients and instead focus on being responsible to our patients by collaborating with them to develop a diabetes self-management program that helps them meet their goals.

3

I let patients make all of their own decisions and medication adjustments. Does that mean that my practice is based on patient empowerment?

 Tip

Part of the definition of empowerment is helping patients take responsibility for their own diabetes care. However, the word "let" implies permission. Only the person who is responsible for decisions can give permission to another person to make them. As educators, we are not responsible for our patients' decisions, only the information and support we provide to help them make those choices. Use of the word "let" implies that as educators we have some control over our patients' behavior. This belief is an illusion. When our patients leave our office, they are in control of their behavior. They can choose to follow our recommendations or not; they are in control.

Although the approach you describe can help patients become more responsible, the true measure of empowerment is in your belief about whose responsibility it is to make decisions.

4

I saw the term "health belief model" in an article I was reading. Can you explain what it is?

 Tip

This model states that health-related behavior is a function of certain beliefs in key areas. The areas include perceived severity and susceptibility to the illness and perceived benefits and barriers to following health recommendations. The model also addresses beliefs related to cues to action and self-efficacy. In the case of diabetes, the health belief model would suggest that the self-management behavior of patients with diabetes could largely be explained by

- how severe they believe diabetes to be
- how susceptible they believe they are to the complications of diabetes
- their beliefs about the benefits of rigorous blood glucose control
- their beliefs about the barriers to implementing an intensive self-management plan

The model would also suggest that environmental factors (i.e., cues to action) that trigger certain behaviors combined with self-efficacy (i.e., their belief in their ability to carry out important self-management behaviors) are also important. Educators who use this model would assess and address each of the key domains of the health belief model.

5

I heard a psychologist mention self-determination theory during a presentation on behavior change. Can you explain this theory?

 Tip

Self-determination theory is based on the recognition that people are required to self-regulate a variety of behaviors that are important but not inherently interesting. Diabetes self-management is a perfect example of such behavior. The theory goes on to assert that patient motivation is a key variable in their ability to initiate and maintain such behaviors. This theory asserts that when patients are internally motivated (i.e., doing something because they believe it's important for their own health and well-being) as opposed to externally motivated (i.e., doing something in order to please a health care professional), they are more likely to initiate and sustain that behavior. Self-determination theory also recognizes that self-efficacy or competence is an important component of the ability to maintain such behaviors.

This theory encourages diabetes educators to support the internalization of motivation so that patients can engage in challenging diabetes self-management behaviors over the long term. Educators can help patients internalize their motivation by asking them questions such as, "What's important to you?" or "What do you want?" or "How do you feel about that?"

6

I heard a colleague of mine say she uses motivational interviewing. Can you tell me what this technique is?

 Tip

Motivational interviewing is a structured approach for helping people recognize and address problems, including behavior change. This approach is based on the recognition that the responsibility for change rests with the individual who is actually carrying out the change.

The five principles of motivational interviewing are

- express empathy
- develop discrepancies
- avoid argumentation
- roll with resistance
- support self-efficacy

The first is the use of empathy, or the warm acceptance of the other person to help create a climate conducive to discussing and implementing behavior changes. The second is the need to focus on discrepancies. For diabetes patients, this might mean a discussion of the discrepancy between their self-management behaviors and their overall commitment to preventing complications and a discussion of the consequences of that discrepancy. Third, although focusing on discrepancies is recommended in motivational interviewing, judgments, arguments, and conflict should be avoided. It would not be in keeping with this model for a diabetes educator to try to convince a patient to change a particular behavior when the patient does not see the need. Fourth, motivational interviewing also recommends that the educator not directly confront patients' resistance to change but rather help them consider new information that may result in a new perspective.

6

Tip *Continued*

For example, a patient who says that complications are inevitable might benefit from a brief summary of the findings of the Diabetes Complications and Control Trial (DCCT) and United Kingdom Prospective Diabetes Study (UKPDS). The final principle, as in other behavior change theories, is the importance of supporting the patient's self-efficacy.

I've heard about the stages of change model, but I'm not sure I understand it. Can you explain this model?

 Tip

The stages of change model is based on the concept that patients are in different stages regarding their readiness to change any particular behavior. The five stages described in this model are

- precontemplation
- contemplation
- preparation
- action
- maintenance

In the first stage, precontemplation, a person is not thinking about changing the target behavior in the foreseeable future. The second stage is contemplation, where the person is thinking about changing the behavior but has not yet made a commitment to change. The third stage is preparation, where the person is planning to make a change in the near future. The fourth stage is action, when the person changes his or her behavior. The fifth stage is maintenance, where the person works to maintain the new behavior and avoid relapse to the previous behavior.

The stages of change model recommends assessing the patient's readiness to change a particular behavior and then tailoring the intervention to match. For example, you might ask, "Have you thought about increasing your level of physical activity to improve your blood glucose control?" The answer to that question would help you understand at which stage the patient is relative to exercise.

The underlying notion is that people change when they are ready to change and not before. It is important to understand a patient's interest in or motivation to change a particular behavior before discussing strategies or plans to change that behavior.

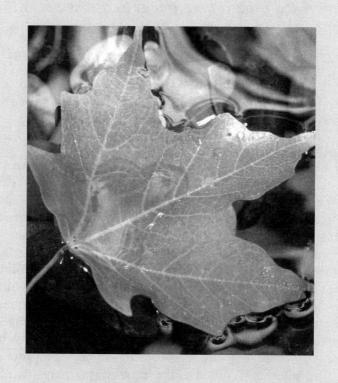

ASSESSMENT

7

I am having a hard time trying to assess patients in all the recommended psychosocial/educational domains such as stress, readiness to change, and family support. Any suggestions?

 Tip

Many assessments are designed to be comprehensive so that you do not miss anything in each domain. However, the cost is that you end up asking a lot of questions that do not produce much useful information. An alternative approach is to ask the patient to identify the critical information. Begin by asking patients to tell you a little bit about what they consider their major problem with diabetes and then ask them how they usually go about solving problems and gathering information. If you ask a few open-ended questions, there is a very high likelihood that patients will provide you with the key information you need to make sure that your education is relevant and tailored to them. For example, rather than giving patients a list of barriers and asking them to check off those that apply, ask, "What are your biggest barriers in managing your diabetes the way you want to?" Because these questions may require some thought, many educators find it helpful to send assessment questions to patients ahead of time and discuss their answers when they arrive.

8

My patients often call to discuss the barriers they are encountering as they try to change their behavior. How can I briefly do a thorough assessment of a problem over the phone?

 Tip

Using the process below will give you a framework for gathering information and making a plan.

S – Subjective data (feelings, tone, level of distress, other issues)

O – Objective data (sex, SMBG, insulin doses, activity, food eaten, etc.)

A – Assessment or presumptive diagnosis

P – Plan/implementation/evaluation

It has been said that 80% of communication is nonverbal. Because you cannot see the patients and get feedback from their facial expression and body language, you are at a disadvantage. You will need to rely on your listening skills to assess the tone of voice, sense of urgency, and level of distress that the caller is experiencing.

Use a focused interview to assess the problem. The following questions might be helpful:

- What is the concern? What are your symptoms?
- How long has this been a concern? How has it developed?
- What is your current regimen (insulin dose, meal plan, activity)?
- What have you tried to do to correct the problem/symptoms?
- Has anything made it better or worse?

9

How can I tell if my patients can afford the supplies and medications they need to take care of their diabetes?

 Tip

Caring for diabetes is expensive, and some people have a hard time paying for the supplies. As a first step, ask assessment questions such as the following:

- Has caring for your diabetes created any financial problems for you?
- Do you ever have a problem paying for your diabetes supplies?
- Does your insurance cover the cost of your supplies and medications?

However, remember that many patients are hesitant to admit that they are having financial problems.

There are also some clues to look for. For example, if patients stop monitoring their blood glucose, or if their blood pressure, once controlled, has started to rise, cost may be an issue. At that point, you can ask patients why they are monitoring less or why their blood pressure is starting to rise. You can also ask if they are having difficulty paying for the strips or the medications. If the lack of money is the reason, they are often relieved that you asked these questions, especially if you offer resources that can help. Keep in mind that the loss of a job, the changing economy, or competing financial priorities can affect patients who could previously afford their supplies and medications.

10

Some of my patients seem to accept their diabetes fairly quickly, whereas others take longer. How can I assess how well patients are adapting?

 Tip

Psychologists call these stages of adaptation. Initially, most patients are shocked and may deny that they have a serious illness. Over time, patients often experience other stages such as anger, depression, blame, resignation, and finally acceptance. Not everyone goes through all of these stages or in that order. The feelings can come and go. In addition, patients may experience times when they go back to earlier stages, for example, if they need to initiate insulin therapy or they develop a complication.

One way to assess how patients are adapting to their illness is to ask two questions: "How did you feel when you first learned that you had diabetes?" and "How do you feel now about having diabetes?" You can also have patients draw a timeline and record significant events in their experiences with diabetes. Ask patients to then identify how they were feeling at the time of each event. Both of these strategies can give you some insight into the patient's frame of mind and also helps patients reflect on how they are feeling about their diabetes at this point in time. Some patients are surprised to see that they have made considerable progress, whereas others learn that they have remained at the same stage.

The purpose is not to move patients from one stage to another. Patients move from one stage to another naturally when they are ready to do so. The purpose is to help them think about their feelings and things that they could do to begin to move toward acceptance.

B Bonus

My patients vary in the degree to which they accept responsibility for their diabetes self-management. Can you give me some ideas about how to assess this?

 Tip

Listen to how your patients talk about their diabetes. Statements such as, "If only my wife would cook the right things . . ." or "If only my job was less stressful . . ." indicate that these patients believe that their diabetes management is largely outside of their control. The key word is "if" because it puts the responsibility on situations or people other than themselves.

Statements such as, "I'm trying not to eat so much, but I get so hungry!" or "I really am trying, but it's so discouraging when I don't see results," can mean they have begun to accept responsibility for their diabetes but are still struggling to live with it effectively. The key word is "but." The first part of the statement acknowledges responsibility, and the second part absolves them from it.

When patients say things such as, "If I don't do it, no one else can do it for me," or "I need to exercise more, so I'm going to schedule time to walk during lunchtime," they have accepted responsibility for their own self-care. The use of unqualified "I" statements is the key.

Keep in mind that patients cannot be forced to accept responsibility. Diabetes is a lifelong disease, and how a patient lives with it is a dynamic process affected by many things. For example, loss of family support, starting on insulin, or the onset of a complication can make the responsibility of diabetes self-management seem overwhelming. Knowing where patients are in that dynamic process can guide you in helping them reflect on what they need to do to make their life with diabetes more manageable.

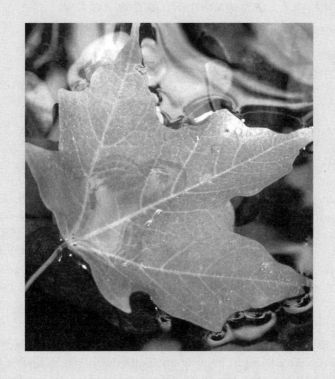

DEALING WITH EMOTION

11

Sometimes I get uncomfortable when my patients express strong feelings of anxiety, anger, or resentment about their diabetes. I don't know how to respond. Any suggestions?

 Tip

Negative emotions are a diabetes educator's best friend. This may seem like an odd thing to say, given how many of us are uncomfortable when others express strong negative emotions. However, it is neither possible nor desirable to "solve" (i.e., get rid of) our patients' negative emotions. Emotions need to be expressed and explored. When we become clear on that point, we can begin to encourage our patients to express such emotions without feeling responsible for making them feel better. One of the things that usually becomes clear is that having an opportunity to express one's emotions to a nonjudgmental and interested listener is therapeutic.

Emotions are the fuel for the engine of behavior change. If we want to maximize the likelihood of helping our patients change behavior, then we can ask them what they are most unhappy or upset about. Patients are more likely to engage in problem-solving and behavior change regarding issues about which they feel strongly. They are unlikely to invest in issues that are important to a diabetes educator but not important to them. The first step is allowing patients to express their emotions freely without any judgment or attempts to make them feel better. When patients have had an adequate opportunity to explore and express their emotions, they will usually be ready to discuss options for improving the situation.

12

When my patients say negative things about their diabetes I want to help them feel better, but I'm not sure how to do it. What do you suggest?

 Tip

It's tempting to try to make patients feel better. However, the motivation for trying to make others feel better often comes from our own discomfort with what they are feeling. We usually do this by putting a positive spin on the situation. For example, we might say, "Oh, it isn't so bad once you know how to handle it," or "Things are never as bad as they seem." However, such responses usually make the person feel worse. These types of comments dismiss the patient's feelings, confirm his or her perception that no one understands, and can add to feelings of failure.

Think about what you would find helpful if you told a friend about how badly you felt about a serious problem you were facing. Most of us want someone to listen and help us gain insight into the issue or situation. Statements such as, "It sounds as if caring for diabetes is a struggle for you. What is hardest for you right now?" or "It must be difficult managing your work schedule, family life, and diabetes every day," validates the patient's feelings, shows respect, and provides the patient with the opportunity to further explore and reflect on his or her feelings. Such responses also let patients know that their feelings are not unusual and that they are not alone. After having a chance to thoroughly explore and express negative feelings, most patients are ready to think about what they could do to improve things for themselves and take action.

13

I get uncomfortable and feel badly if patients cry during a session. What can I do to keep them from getting upset when I ask them about living with diabetes?

 Tip

The first question to ask yourself is, "Why do I feel badly when patients cry?" Do you feel uncomfortable if patients laugh during a session? Crying is an appropriate way to express and release emotions. It is a sign that patients trust you enough to show their feelings.

Diabetes educators sometimes feel uncomfortable when patients react with tears because we think we "made them cry" and/or our job is to make our patients feel better. But diabetes is a difficult, life-changing disease. Tears are a normal response to sad and painful facts of life. There is nothing you can say that will change the reality of diabetes, and attempts to minimize it (e.g., "Don't worry, everything will be okay") devalue patients' experiences.

You may feel uncomfortable because you don't know what to do when a patient cries. Usually, silence and perhaps a caring touch are all you need to do. There is nothing you need to say other than to reassure the patient that crying is an acceptable and usual part of living with diabetes. Crying is part of the grieving process. The tears patients shed brings them closer to living peacefully with diabetes.

14

I seem to encounter a lot of angry patients. What can I do to help them get over their anger?

 Tip

Anger is a fairly common response to a chronic illness, particularly one that affects as many aspects of life as diabetes does. Although it is not possible to simply "get patients over" their anger, you can help patients to examine their feelings and how they affect their behavior.

One of the things you can do is acknowledge and reflect those feelings in statements to patients by asking questions such as, "Are you feeling angry about _____?" Such a question lets patients know that you are listening to them. Adding a question such as, "Can you tell me more about that?" can help patients better express those feelings to you.

We prefer to use questions because helping patients identify and discuss what they are specifically angry about lets them know that you are interested in hearing more about their feelings. Simply making the assertion, "You sound angry," may sound patronizing to the patient and may diminish rather than increase communication. Although it may help some patients to know that anger is a natural response to an illness such as diabetes, be careful not to minimize the intensity of the patient's personal experience with anger by only telling him or her that it is "normal to feel that way."

Anger is a negative emotion that can be used positively as a way of fighting back. It provides the energy for some patients to take control of their diabetes once they are able to recognize and channel this powerful emotion.

15

A *lot of my patients seem to feel guilty about having diabetes or getting complications. What can I say to help decrease their feelings of guilt?*

 Tip

Guilt is a common feeling that many patients experience. It is especially common among parents of children with diabetes as they try to find out why their child was affected in that way. Guilt is generally not useful because it is often related to past activities, and those cannot be changed. Guilt can cause patients to become stuck considering, "What I should have done," rather than coping with how things are now.

Although it is tempting to tell patients that they should not feel guilty or that they may have developed the complications of diabetes even if they had done everything they could, neither of those responses is particularly helpful. If you think about times when you have felt guilty, others telling you that you shouldn't feel that way probably did not change your view and may have caused you to feel devalued and misunderstood.

A more useful strategy is to reflect guilty feelings and the cause of them back to the patient. For example, you may say, "Are you feeling guilty because you didn't do some things to take care of yourself?" Once the patient has had the opportunity to express those feelings, it may be useful to acknowledge that although we cannot change the past, we can learn from it. Ask what the person has learned from this experience that might be applied in the future. You can also ask if there are ways the guilty feelings could be channeled in a more positive way in the future or if it would be helpful for you to provide more information about the area of concern.

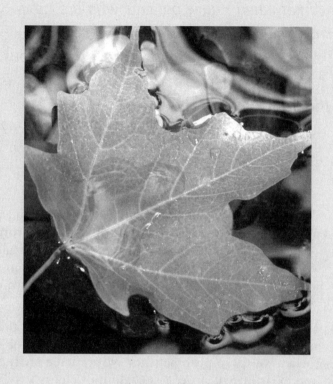

CHOOSING TO CHANGE

16

Sometimes when I have patients who are close to making a big change or a significant breakthrough in their diabetes care, I get anxious and try to move them along. I suspect that this is not the most useful thing to do, but I have trouble resisting the temptation. Any suggestions?

 Tip

It's very easy to see why this situation provides such a temptation. You clearly want the best for your patients and are probably worried that they may not go the last step towards the kind of change or breakthrough for which you think they are ready. This may explain your anxiety, especially if you are worried that your patients may not return or might actually relapse if the change doesn't happen now.

In such situations, it can be helpful to remind ourselves that breakthroughs and changes have to be made *by* patients and can't be made *for* them. Also, when we try to push patients, we are more likely to create resistance than to facilitate change. You could try to focus the discussion on the patient's perceptions of what else needs to happen for change to occur. To help patients understand what they themselves want and need rather than focusing on what the educator hopes will happen, use questions such as:

- What has to happen for you to make the final step to achieve the long-term goal you set?
- Do you need more time? Are you ready to make a commitment?
- Is there something holding you back?
- What do you think a next step would be for you? How can I help you?

17

What do I do when my patient says, "Just tell me what to do"?

 Tip

Being responsible for managing an illness is a new concept for some patients and may be overwhelming, particularly early in the diagnosis. Patients want an expert to tell them how to manage diabetes the "right" way. By giving them a plan in response to that statement, you are meeting the need they have identified.

As you develop the plan, try to engage patients as much as possible in refining the plan. For example, ask them about the foods they enjoy and activities in which they participate. Let them know that as they put a plan developed by someone else in place, they are likely to get frustrated on days when the plan isn't quite right or when they get tired of living with someone else's ideas. This type of interaction begins the process for helping patients assume greater responsibility for designing a self-management plan of their own. Most patients are not content to use the same plan on a long-term basis, and they may be tempted to stop taking care of their diabetes. If they have this experience, let them know that you are available to work with them to create a plan designed to fit their lives.

18

I've heard that patients often make decisions based on costs and benefits. How can I help them to think about the costs and benefits of their diabetes care decisions?

 Tip

Most of the important decisions we make are based on weighing positives and negatives. Every change we contemplate has both costs and benefits. We often make changes in our lives when the benefits of making the change outweigh the costs or the negative aspects for keeping things the same.

One useful activity to help patients think about costs and benefits is to write the words "costs" and "benefits" on the board and put a line between them. Then ask the individual or group to identify costs and benefits for decisions they have to make or a common issue in diabetes care, such as tight glucose control or weight loss. Ask the person or group to brainstorm and simply write the answers. Do not attempt to minimize costs or praise benefits.

Once the list is complete, ask the group to tell you their thoughts about the list. One common occurrence is that patients identify that many of the costs are short term, whereas the benefits are long term. This is an important insight because much of what is done for diabetes care on a day-to-day basis has great future benefits and may have daily costs.

Then ask patients to think about whether the costs are worth the benefits in their own lives. Point out that this is a personal decision that no one else can make for them because no one else is an expert on their lives.

I find that even when patients clearly need insulin to manage their blood glucose levels, they are often resistant. How can I help them?

 Tip

Taking insulin is a big step for many patients and one that many patients dread. Although resistance is a common reaction, the reasons why patients resist insulin therapy are varied. Some patients have seen others develop complications from diabetes, such as amputations or impotence, or even die shortly after going on insulin. Others may be feeling pressure from family and friends not to go on insulin because of how it will affect their lifestyle. They may worry that they will lose flexibility or be restricted from travel or other activities. For others, it is a sign that diabetes is truly a serious disease or perhaps they can no longer keep their diabetes secret from others. Insulin may represent aging, worsening disease, loss of independence, or failure if they are no longer able to manage their diabetes with meal planning and activity. Or, the patient may be afraid of needles or concerned about the hassle of insulin administration.

The first step is to assess the reason for that particular patient's resistance. Questions such as, "Why don't you want to go on insulin?" or "What does going on insulin mean to you?" can help you and your patients figure out why insulin is an issue for them. This can then guide you in providing the appropriate information or support so that the patient can make a decision that will work for him or her.

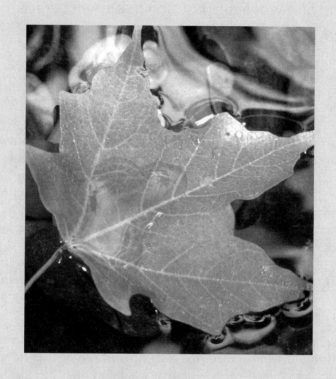

MOTIVATION

19

Some of my patients just don't seem motivated.
What can I do to motivate them?

 Tip

You can't motivate your patients because they are already motivated. But, they are motivated to accomplish their own goals. When educators ask how they can motivate patients, they usually mean, "How can I motivate my patients to do what I want them to do?" Although you might be able to provide some short-term motivation by reinforcing behaviors so that patients make changes in order to win your approval, over the long term, this strategy usually causes more problems than it solves. First, you are accepting responsibility to provide a patient's ongoing motivation, which will eventually become a burden for you. Second, patients are unlikely to stay motivated to engage in sometimes difficult self-management behaviors simply to maintain the approval of health care professionals.

Discovering what motivates the patient now is critical. If a patient is motivated in a direction that you consider unhealthy, it is important to understand what needs of the patient are being met by that behavior. Although patients may make unwise choices, the needs they are trying to meet are almost always valid. The likelihood that they will change their behavior is very small unless we can help them discover other strategies for meeting the same needs. For example, rather than trying to convince a patient of the value of blood glucose monitoring, we might say, "Help me understand your reluctance to do blood glucose monitoring." We might learn that the patient's refusal is a means to show the health care professional that the patient is in charge of his or her own life. Such a patient can usually be helped to find more effective ways of expressing his or her valid need for autonomy. In this example, communicating openly and assertively with health care professionals would be a more effective and less harmful strategy than simply resisting their recommendations. The key is discovering what is motivating the patient now, accepting the validity of the needs he or she is trying to meet, and helping that patient decide if the strategy he or she is using is effective.

20

If I had diabetes I would do everything possible to take care of myself. Why are so many of my patients unwilling to give 100% to their diabetes care?

 Tip

To learn the answer to that question, it might help to walk a mile in their shoes. One of the activities we have used in training programs for health professionals is to ask participants to follow a simulated self-management regimen for three to five days in order to experience the tasks that people with diabetes do every day. We asked them to take two saline injections a day, check their blood glucose levels four times a day and record the results, eat a 1,200-calorie diet at appropriate times, check their feet daily, and exercise 30 minutes per day. They were surprised at how hard it was, how often they "failed," the intrusiveness of diabetes, and the intensity of their feelings of anger and loss of control over their lives even though it was only for a few days.

You might try an experiment such as this alone, or better still, with some of your colleagues. You could carry it further by adding the cost of two or three diabetes medications (e.g., a lipid-lowering drug and an ACE inhibitor) into your budget. When you exercise, be mindful that your blood glucose shouldn't be too high or too low before you start. You could also imagine having high blood glucose, making frequent (and sometimes inconvenient) visits to the bathroom, having a thirst that is impossible to quench, and needing to look for yet another pair of glasses to help your blurred vision. Imagine being so tired that you have to force yourself to do your usual activities and experiencing the despair of seeing a high number on your monitor when you have done everything you know how to do. Write down your feelings about your experiences or talk about them with your colleagues.

Even though we cannot truly know what it is like to have diabetes unless we develop it ourselves, following a simulated regimen can significantly deepen our appreciation of the many challenges faced by people living with diabetes every day.

21

I get frustrated when I tell patients that I need to see their blood glucose records in order to take the best possible care of their diabetes, but they still don't want to test. What can I say to convince them?

 Tip

Most of us are not very motivated to cause ourselves pain for another person. A lot of people don't like to check their blood glucose, for a variety of reasons. As diabetes educators, our job is to provide an environment where patients can examine the cost-benefit ratio of a variety of self-care behaviors, including monitoring.

Instead of asking patients to test a prescribed number of times per day, try asking, "How do you use the information that you get from testing your blood?" or "How often do you need to check your blood glucose to get the information you need to manage your diabetes?" If patients are not using the monitoring information in their daily life, then it's not surprising that they are not interested in checking their blood glucose. After all, monitoring can be expensive, painful, and unpleasant.

The ideas we convey with the words we use may also have an effect. The word "test" has the connotation of a judgment—good, bad, pass, or fail. Try using the words "check" or "monitor" when talking about doing the readings.

If the blood glucose readings are rarely in range, rarely change, or make the patient feel like a failure, then it is easy for them to skip. Presenting the concept of blood glucose readings as data needed to make informed decisions may be helpful. Remind patients that their blood glucose level is not a measure of their worth as a person; it's simply information that can be used to help them make self-management decisions.

22

It's hard for me to understand my obese patients. You'd think they would want to lose weight for their diabetes, their general health, and their looks. How can I help them?

 Tip

There is a lot we don't know about obesity. Many health professionals still fail to recognize that obesity is not a character flaw, but a chronic illness with a genetic/physiological basis. Research is being done to help us understand the various genetic and cellular components of obesity, but we currently don't have highly effective treatments for the condition. Although eating less and exercising more helps patients lose weight, most people have difficulty beginning or sustaining those behaviors, especially if they are trying to make big changes.

People eat for a variety of physical and emotional reasons. Many of us eat when we are blessed, stressed, or depressed. Food often represents caring and comfort. There is nothing wrong with eating as a coping device, it is just that most of us don't use that device very wisely.

Many overweight patients with diabetes expect to be judged harshly by society and especially by health professionals. They may appear defensive or negative. It is important that these patients feel accepted and respected. Most overweight adults have tried many "diets" and may have lost and regained hundreds of pounds. They may have unrealistic expectations and believe that they are failures if they do not achieve or maintain substantial weight loss.

Rather than assuming that such patients don't know the benefits of weight loss, ask if they are interested in a nutrition referral and in working on their weight. If they are not interested, focus on meal planning to manage blood glucose. This feels less judgmental and often results in modest weight loss.

22

Tip *Continued*

If patients are interested in losing weight, rather than focusing on an ideal weight, let them know that a 10–15% weight loss has been shown to reduce insulin resistance. Help them to create a meal plan they can *use* rather than *follow*. It is also helpful for patients to choose goals that focus on behaviors rather than pounds. The scales don't always recognize our efforts, and weight loss can be slow. A behavioral approach helps them to make changes in their eating habits that can be sustained so that weight loss can be maintained.

23

Some of my patients seem to accept high blood glucose as normal. I have talked with them over and over about the risk of complications, but they have a fatalistic attitude. How can I help them to understand that there is something they can do about diabetes?

 Tip

Statements such as, "My blood glucose has been high for a long time, and I haven't had any problems," or "I feel fine when my blood glucose is high, so I'm not going to worry about it," are frustrating for us as educators. We have seen the negative consequences of this way of thinking, so we are concerned. We often respond by becoming more vigorous in our efforts to try to convince our patients otherwise and to make suggestions for changing behavior. This usually makes the problem worse by increasing denial.

One approach is to let the patient know that you are concerned. Statements such as, "I am very concerned about you because of what I know and what I have seen," or "I feel frustrated because it seems that I am more concerned more about your diabetes than you are," may open the door to a fruitful conversation. But the reality is that we can't force people to care nor can we convince them to change. All we can do is offer information and our support and be available when and if they decide the time is right to work on their diabetes care.

24

Are there some behavioral techniques that you can recommend? No matter what I say, I just can't seem to get my patients to change.

 Tip

That's not surprising because it really isn't possible to get another person to change.

Think about the changes and choices you have made in your own life. Did anyone get you to change or did you look at the situation and decide that the benefits for making the change outweighed the costs? A common response to that question is, "I just needed to make up my mind to do it." Others can inform, inspire, and support us, but lasting change comes from within.

People with diabetes make decisions the same way. They make choices and changes based on feelings, information, costs and benefits, and their belief in their ability to reach their goals. Change occurs naturally when the conditions are right. The purpose of diabetes education is to provide patients with the information they need to make informed choices and select their own goals and then to provide the skills and strategies they need to make the changes to accomplish their goals.

25

I find it very frustrating that my patients don't do everything they can to take care of themselves. I sometimes think it is a good idea to scare them into taking care of themselves. Is that a useful thing to do?

 Tip

Scare tactics are generally not useful when working with most patients. In general, scare tactics tend to increase denial and guilt rather than decrease negative behaviors. Even if patients do make changes based on scare tactics, they are generally short lived. Most people respond more actively to messages of hope rather than fear.

Knowing about diabetes complications is part of being an informed person with diabetes, and it is our responsibility as health professionals to provide that information to our patients. However, such information is more effective when it is provided along with strategies that will help patients prevent or detect complications. For example, you can let patients know that diabetes care today is a bad news/good news situation. The bad news is that complications can and do occur in spite of everything we, and they, do. The good news is that more is known about preventing and treating complications then ever before. By becoming active participants in their own care, patients can help to prevent the complications or find them early when they can be treated more easily.

26

I've heard other educators talk about active listening. What exactly is active listening?

 Tip

Active listening means using communication skills that further the patient's exploration and expression of their experience of living with diabetes. It involves listening attentively, asking questions, and making statements that encourage the patient to discover the heart of the issue. Indicate that you are listening by using statements that summarize and reflect back what you've heard, such as, "So you're saying . . ." or "If I heard correctly, you're feeling . . ."

Active listening is a learned skill that improves with practice. The use of rhetorical questions is not an example of attentive/active listening because these questions are generally perceived as criticism or interrogation, for example, "Don't you think that you could put a bit more effort into trying to control your diabetes?" Using rhetorical questions is an indirect way of expressing an opinion without accepting responsibility for doing so. On the other hand, questions and reflective statements convey the educator's interest and compassion, which patients experience as a validation of their self-worth. Often the most useful part of a discussion facilitated through active listening is the insight that patients accrue from listening to their own stories.

Our role is to create an environment where those stories are nurtured, welcomed, and valued. Active listening often helps patients explore and express the emotions that provide their motivation for behavior change.

27

I've learned that sustaining change is hard. How can I help my patients stay motivated to maintain changes in their behavior over the long term?

 Tip

Diabetes self-management involves making behavior changes that many patients find difficult to sustain. Changes in eating behavior and physical activity are two notable examples. The role that we can play as educators in helping patients sustain behavior changes is crucial.

Many people begin a new behavior with great enthusiasm, but over time that enthusiasm often wanes, and they return to their previous behaviors. Sometimes, the press of daily life pushes diabetes self-management into the background. We can help our patients by calling their attention to their diabetes self-management plan and helping them reflect on the contribution it makes to their life. To help them reflect on the changes they made, you can ask, "What impact did those changes have on your life and your diabetes care?" or "What was your original motivation for making those changes?" This moves their self-management behavior and their motivation back into the psychological foreground.

Behavior change is an ongoing process and is one of the reasons why it is important to think about diabetes education as a long-term endeavor. The notion that patients will simply acquire knowledge, change behavior, and then sustain those changes is patently naive. We can make a significant contribution to our patients by helping them remember and rediscover the motivation that brought about the original changes in their behavior.

D Bonus

I want my patients to learn to speak up and become more assertive consumers of diabetes care. What would you suggest?

 Tip

A good way to begin is by helping them understand the nature and purpose of assertive communication. Assertiveness is most useful in situations where people feel threatened, anxious, or uncomfortable. For example, expressing dissatisfaction or disagreement to a health professional is uncomfortable for most patients. People often respond to anxiety-provoking situations in one of two ways. The first is by getting angry and blaming or criticizing the perceived source of anxiety, that is, the professional. Others take the opposite approach and hide their discomfort, become passive, and do not address the issue at all. These are examples of the fight and flight response to a perceived threat. Assertive communication lies between these two ineffective extremes. In assertive communication we take responsibility for feelings and behavior. When communicating assertively, we state openly what we think, feel, and want, while acknowledging that others may think, feel, and want differently than us. We recognize that each of us has a right to our views. Problem-solving discussions and negotiations then proceed from positions of responsibility and mutual respect. You might help your patients practice "I" statements, for example, "I think," "I want," "I feel" (as opposed to, "You make me feel"). Making "I" statements is a first step in communicating assertively.

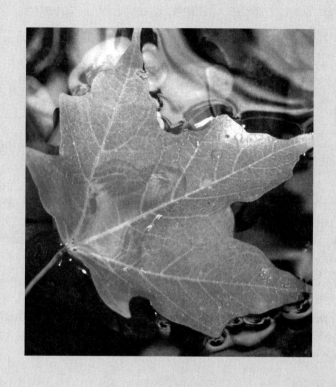

ATTITUDES,

BELIEFS, AND

VALUES

28

__W__hat do attitudes, beliefs, and values have to do with diabetes education?

 Tip

Our values and beliefs are important components of our attitudes. Our attitudes have a great deal to do with how we behave.

There are times when we view our patients' behavior as irrational. It is hard for us to understand why having knowledge about diabetes and its care isn't enough to help them make changes in their behavior. Often, this is because their attitudes, beliefs, and values have more influence over their behavior than the knowledge they have gained.

You cannot change another person's attitudes, beliefs, or values. However, you can facilitate a powerful learning experience by helping patients reflect on the effect of their attitudes on their behavior and whether their attitudes are helping or hindering their efforts to achieve the outcomes that they want.

I find that some patients have a very bad attitude about their diabetes. What can I do to help those patients look at diabetes more positively?

 Tip

Every person with diabetes responds differently to hearing about and living with diabetes. Even when the diagnosis and treatment are the same, some patients always view diabetes as a disaster, whereas others are able to live more peacefully with it over time.

The words patients choose are often powerful indicators of their attitudes and feelings. If they tend to use particular words, you can ask them to describe the word or phrase further. For example you could say, "I notice that you always describe diabetes as a horrible disease. Can you tell me more about that?" Another approach is to ask patients to choose a word from a list to describe their diabetes. You can make up your own list from words you hear patients use often, or use a list such as disaster, burden, problem, challenge, and opportunity. Be sure the list includes a range of attitudes. Ask the patient to then describe why he or she chose that word. You can also ask the patient to describe how that feeling helps or hinders his or her self-care efforts.

The point of this activity is not to change the patient's attitude. It is meant to help patients examine how their attitude is affecting their behavior and their ability to live with diabetes. Trying to get someone to change his or her attitude usually produces resistance. Patients need to express and explore their attitudes so that they can change when they are ready to do so.

30

I understand that I need to help patients clarify their values about diabetes. How can I do that?

 Tip

Our values are the things that we believe in and cherish and are most important to us in our lives. They have a very strong influence on our behavior, even though we may not often think about our values.

For example, most people state that they want to be healthy and independent. Health is a value for them. However, if the things that they need to do to be healthy are not compatible with other values (e.g., their role in the family), then conflict occurs. Even though they value health, other more immediate values may take precedence.

A simple way to help patients clarify their values is to provide a structure for patients to identify, examine, and prioritize the values in their life. It can be as simple as an open-ended statement such as, "My most important goal in caring for my diabetes is . . ." Another idea is to ask participants to list the five most important things in their life in order of priority and then to identify where diabetes fits on the list. The idea is not to change or judge their values, but to help them examine how their values influence their behavior and self-care efforts.

31

A lot of my patients respond negatively when I suggest that diabetes is something that they need to learn to "cope" with. Is there another word I can use?

 Tip

A lot of people respond negatively to the word "cope." Coping often seems passive, as if you should just accept whatever comes your way. But the true meaning of the word is not passive at all. When we are confronted with difficulties in our lives, we can either solve them or learn to cope with them. Diabetes is a problem that does not go away. It cannot be solved. When we have problems that we cannot solve, we need to learn to cope with them. Coping is a way of dealing with situations that do not go away.

It may help if you explain coping as an active process. Part of coping is taking charge of your diabetes and learning to live with it peacefully and effectively. Point out that patients can make decisions about how actively they are involved in their care, their goals, and their behaviors. Coping means that they are doing all they can to take charge of their future. It also implies coming to a psychological peace with diabetes. Because our feelings greatly influence our behaviors, coming to peace with diabetes also has an effect on outcomes.

It may be useful to ask patients what the word coping means to them. If the words are relatively passive, ask if they have other words that they use to describe how they live with diabetes. You can also ask if they have thought about the decisions they make and the ways they reflect on and deal with their feelings as a way of coping. These strategies can help patients take a more positive view of coping.

32

My patients seem to respond negatively when I talk about "controlling their diabetes." Is there other language I can use?

 Tip

Many patients don't like when we refer to "controlling their diabetes." Although as health professionals we know that we are referring to their blood glucose or A1C, patients often believe that we are talking about their self-control. They view our statement as a judgment of their total efforts in managing their diabetes.

Rather than using the word "control" or the phrase "out of control," simply describe what you mean. For example, when looking at a logbook, you can say, "I see that your blood glucose is out of the target range before dinner almost every day," or "It looks like you are having quite a few blood glucose reactions before lunch." These statements are not only clearer, but they are also generally perceived as more factual and less judgmental.

33

I've had patients with one or more complications ask, "Why would God punish me like this?" I have no idea how to respond to such a question. Do you have any suggestions?

 Tip

Keep in mind that it is very unlikely that the patient expects you to have an answer to this question. Rather, the patient is expressing feelings of grief and is trying to integrate this experience into his or her particular viewpoint.

The major contribution of a diabetes educator in these situations is to actively listen to patients as they explore and express their feelings about such issues. Start with asking, "Do you think God is punishing you?" Your next strategy might be to listen, as your patients struggle to come to grips with this new development. Asking clarifying questions in response to their statements will help them to reflect and will let patients know you're interested. At the end of such an encounter, let patients know that you are there for them. It might also be helpful to ask them if there are pastors, priests, rabbis, or ministers that could help them sort out this aspect of their experience.

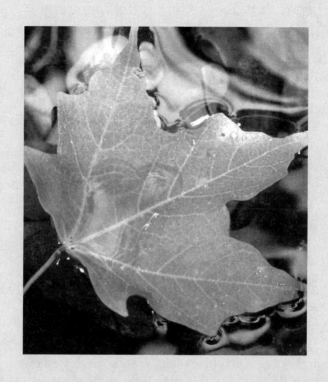

GOAL-SETTING

34

I've heard that goal-setting is an important part of my role as an educator. How can I set goals with patients?

 Tip

Goal-setting is a proven strategy that patients can use to make changes in their behavior. To help patients set goals, break the process down into steps. The five steps for setting goals are

- identify the problem
- explore feelings
- set goals
- make a plan
- evaluate the result

Although this may seem like a long process, each step is critical. If we skip over identifying the problem or feelings, we risk setting a goal to solve a symptom rather than the real problem. Sometimes the real problem is identified only after exploration of the problem initially described by the patient. If we focus only on the problem and feelings and don't identify an action to take, patients may remain stuck on a particular issue. If you can't get through all five steps in one visit, you can always end the discussion by asking the patient to think more about the process and then begin where you left off at your next visit or telephone contact.

35

I know that I need to set behavioral goals with patients, but when I ask about their goals, they don't seem to know what I am talking about. What are some strategies to use?

 Tip

Although patients may set goals in other areas of their lives, they don't always think of setting goals for their health-related behaviors. One approach is to ask patients a series of questions that will help them think about their diabetes care efforts. Examples of such questions are:

- What is the worst or hardest thing for you about caring for your diabetes?
- Why is that?
- How does dealing with this issue make you feel?
- What would have to change for it to get better?
- In six months, what would you like to have accomplished in this area?
- Are you willing to begin to make some of those changes?
- What are some changes that you can make for that to happen?
- What can you do this week to get started?

36

***W**hat are some strategies I can use to teach my patients how to set specific goals? They tend to choose very big areas on which to work, and it is hard to get specific in a short time.*

 Tip

An easy but effective strategy is to teach patients to ask themselves, "Why?" and "How?" five times. Asking "why" helps the patient to think more specifically about the true nature of the problem that he or she is trying to solve. Because some of the "whys" are often a reaction to our emotional response to a situation, it is also a way of helping patients think about their feelings and how their feelings influence their behavior.

Asking "how" five times helps patients to get very specific about exactly what they will do. It helps the patient to move from goals such as, "I will use my meal plan every day," to a very specific behavioral goal such as, "I will eat one green vegetable at each meal."

Asking how and why are ways to help patients achieve clarity. This is also an effective strategy for helping patients work at their goal attainment.

The following example is from a dialogue that occurred in one of our classes:

Patient: I said I was going to eat more vegetables this week, but I didn't.

Educator: Why?

Patient: My husband cooks, and he doesn't cook vegetables. I bought some, but I didn't fix them.

Educator: Why?

Tip *Continued*

Patient: I don't want to cook two meals. I bought cut up carrots to eat raw, but I didn't.

Educator: Why?

Patient: I didn't want to go in the kitchen.

Educator: Why?

Patient: I lost 20 pounds by staying out of the kitchen, and I'm not going back in there!

Educator: You told me that one of the reasons you wanted to eat more vegetables was to keep the weight off. Given what you learned from this experience, do you have any other thoughts about how you can reach that goal?

Patient: I was thinking I wanted to be more active, the way I was before my grandkids moved in.

Educator: How can you do that?

Patient: Well, I used to take a class, but I can't do that anymore.

Educator: So how do you think you can be more active?

Patient: We go to the park almost every day. We could walk instead of drive. It's about 10 minutes away.

Educator: How do you think that will work for you?

Patient: Well, sometimes I do errands when we leave, but I can walk at least two days this week. I'll try that.

37

When patients reach their goals, should I give lots of positive reinforcement?

 Tip

Most educators learned that providing positive reinforcement helps to promote behavior change. But there are some reasons to rethink this strategy.

When we provide positive reinforcement, we are making a judgment about the patient's behavior. The implication is that because we have the right to praise behavior, we also have the right to criticize behavior. This creates an unequal relationship and distance between the patient and the educator. We take on the role of being the parent or judge.

Almost everyone wants to be liked and wants others to think well of them. When we provide positive reinforcement for what we judge to be positive behaviors, patients may tend to tell us what we want to hear so that we continue to think well of them. An example is when a patient's blood glucose records and A1C levels don't seem to correlate. We may have created the situation where patients feel like they have to give us good values for us to like them or to avoid being "scolded."

One of the reasons educators provide reinforcement is that we sometimes believe that our patients' behaviors are a reflection of our skill as an educator. But patients do not take care of themselves for us. We need to help patients understand that they take care of their diabetes for themselves, not to please others.

Positive reinforcement also creates a situation where our opinion seems more important than that of the patient. If we applaud two pounds of weight loss as a good amount to lose, we negate the patient's disappointment that they haven't met their goal of losing five pounds or the opportunity to learn from a discussion about what went wrong. If we can't tell from our patients' demeanor that they are pleased with their results, we can simply ask what they think about their efforts.

37

Tip *Continued*

Does this mean that you never say anything good to patients? Of course not! Statements such as, "I can see that you are really putting a lot of effort into your diabetes care these days," or "I really appreciate that you keep all of your appointments," helps us recognize the efforts patients make, but not the behaviors. We can celebrate *with* our patients and not *for* our patients.

38

I don't know what to say when patients do not reach their goals. What is a useful response?

 Tip

One approach is to help patients think of their behavior-change efforts as experiments. We use experiments to try new things and to determine if the plan we have developed is a good one. When we work with patients to set goals, we can set the stage by suggesting that they view their behavioral goals as experiments. The goals become an opportunity to see what does and does not work.

One of the reasons behavioral goals are not reached is that we haven't figured out what the real problem is. When a patient hasn't reached his or her goal, ask, "Why not?" or "What got in the way of reaching your goal?" The answers to such questions will help patients choose behaviors that will help them move toward their goal.

It may also help to think about why we find it hard to respond when our patients don't reach their goals. Does some of the discomfort come from our belief that patients who are not successful reflect on our abilities as an educator? Is it because we are uncomfortable when patients express negative emotions? Is it because we want patients to like us so we try to take away any negative feelings they have? In other words, ask yourself why you feel uncomfortable.

Many scientists believe that they learn as much from the experiments that don't work as from those that do. We can help patients learn from both positive and negative experiences. We approach this issue with the idea that there is no such thing as failure, only feedback.

*H*ow do I set goals and make a plan on the phone?

 Tip

Reflecting back to the patient the information you have heard and distilled from your assessment will help patients identify their main issues. Creating a plan involves asking patients what they think they could do to resolve their problem. Usually patients will come up with several things they could try. Sometimes focusing on one step they can work on until they come into the office again is helpful. Having them record what they are doing in their logbook or on a calendar helps them see the progress that they are making toward reaching their goal. Having them fax, e-mail, or call periodically will help them to continue moving forward.

Here are some helpful discussion points:

- What one thing causes you the most difficulty? Shall we start with that?
- Let me make sure that I heard your concern accurately. You are very worried about (summarize what you heard the patient say).
- We have identified four potential solutions. Let's review them so you can decide which to try out.
- Let's take this one step at a time. What is one goal you can focus on until your next visit?

40

I don't know what to do when patients set their blood glucose target too high or too low. Should I try to persuade them to change it?

 Tip

Keep in mind that it is ultimately the patients' right and responsibility to select their own target range. Rather than persuasion, a useful approach is to ask, "Why did you pick that number?" You can then use this information to begin the discussion about their chosen target range.

Asking patients why they selected the target they did may help clarify their feelings or fears about diabetes. Perhaps they have symptoms of hypoglycemia even when their blood glucose is in the normal range. Perhaps they are so afraid of complications they want to keep their blood glucose in or below the normal range all the time. Perhaps they don't know the link between blood glucose levels and complications.

You can then use additional questions to help them clarify if they have chosen a reasonable and achievable target. Questions such as, "Do you think this level is a realistic goal for you at this time?" or "On a scale of one to ten, with ten being the most important, how important is it to you to achieve your target?" can help both you and the patient determine if the target is reasonable.

41

What should I do when my patients choose behavioral strategies or goals that I don't think will make any real difference in their glucose levels or overall health?

 Tip

There are a couple of points to keep in mind in this kind of situation. The first is that patients are much more likely to pursue goals they have chosen for themselves than those suggested by a diabetes educator. So, unless your patients' goals present some risk to their health or well-being, it's probably a mistake to try to change their minds. Rather, it would help to have you and your patients view the goal as an experiment. You might say, "Well, why don't you give it a try and see how things work out." If it turns out that the patient has chosen a goal that doesn't have any demonstrable impact, you and the patient can use that information to select another goal with a higher likelihood of affecting the outcome. Remember, even if the goal didn't have a demonstrable impact on blood glucose control or other metabolic parameters, the patient did demonstrate a willingness and ability to make behavioral changes to improve his or her diabetes care. Acknowledge and support such behavior.

42

*W*hat do I do when patients greet me with a litany of failed goals and high blood glucose because of a variety of family and other problems?

 Tip

The real question is why they feel the need to greet you that way. In the past, many people with diabetes were treated as children and judged harshly if they didn't "do as they were told." If that is what patients anticipate, they may initiate the visit in ways to deflect attention away from themselves and try to diffuse the situation because of how they think you will respond. After all, it is human nature to want to be successful and please people we think are making judgments about us.

We need to provide a safe environment for our patients—one that allows them to focus on what works for them and what doesn't. Agreeing that family and other problems are very stressful validates their feelings of frustration and acknowledges that diabetes is not the only priority in their lives.

If this happens often with particular patients, however, then it is appropriate to discuss the matter frankly. Perhaps they are overwhelmed by the problems in their lives. They may be setting unrealistic goals or ones that are chosen to please you rather than ones that have meaning for them.

This may also be a sign that the patient needs to take a break from setting goals. If the patient is feeling overwhelmed, you may choose to spend the time you have together talking about those issues or coping strategies. If the goals are unrealistic or chosen to please you, then you may want to discuss the importance of the patient's role as a decision-maker.

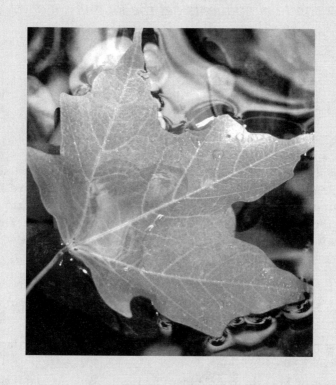

SOCIAL

SUPPORT

43

How can I help patients get the kind of support they need and want?

 Tip

One of the most effective ways is to help them learn to ask for it. People don't always know what kind of support they have available or what kind they want. An example of an activity that will help patients to clarify the support they need and want is described below. This activity works well in a group or individual session, either as a written or spoken activity.

- List behaviors by others that you find helpful and supportive.
- List behaviors by others that you find are not helpful or even hurtful.
- List people in your life from whom you want support: family, friends, and coworkers.
- Describe how the people identified show support and if it is helpful or not.

Now review your lists. If there are behaviors that you would find helpful that are not available to you currently, note the people who you could ask for this type of support. If the behaviors that you are currently encountering are in the "not helpful" category, think about ways you can convey your distress to that person.

If patients are unable to identify sources of support, ask them to brainstorm ideas for supporters outside their current network, or ask if a support group would be helpful for them.

Family members and friends generally want to be helpful and supportive, but they don't always know how. Many patients find that asking their friends and family for what they need and want will take them a long way towards getting that support.

Some of my patients say, "My family is 'on' me all the time." What can I do to help them get the kind of support from their family that they need?

 Tip

Diabetes is a family disease. Changes in the meal plan may affect the whole family, and time spent exercising can mean time away from the family. The diagnosis of diabetes can also be frightening for family members. They can feel helpless, frustrated, and angry. They are usually concerned when they see their loved ones doing something they view as detrimental to their diabetes care and long-term health. In their attempts to be helpful, they can begin to nag and become a drain to the person with diabetes. Assuming the role of the "diabetes police" is usually a response of family members to their own anxiety related to the diabetes. This behavior can also have a negative effect on family dynamics and spread to other aspects of family life.

Although it is useful to understand why families may become "diabetes police," that doesn't mean that their actions are helpful. If the person with diabetes doesn't perceive the behavior as supportive, then it isn't. There are strategies you can provide to patients that can help them to receive the support that they want from family and friends.

- Most people are not well versed in the significant changes that have taken place in diabetes self-management recently. Let the participants know that they can bring family members or friends to classes.

- Discuss the possibility of a support group for families or inviting family members to attend a support group with the person affected by diabetes.

- The best way to get the support you need is to ask for exactly the kind of support you want. Most family members want to be supportive and may not know that their behavior is not helpful.

44

Tip *Continued*

- If patients are uncomfortable about asking for support, you can try practicing the situation with the patient playing one role and you or another member of the group portraying the family member. If support is a common issue for a group, you can ask them to identify and role-play the situation.

- If some patients feel as though they cannot talk to the person, or have tried without success, you might suggest that they compose a letter describing a particular interaction that upset them. The letter can include what both parties could have done to help make a better outcome for all concerned. Ask if they wish to share the letter with that person, or perhaps the act of writing their thoughts down now makes it easier to describe their feelings directly to the person.

45

Some of my patients say they feel very alone. Should I suggest going to a support group?

 Tip

Many people with diabetes feel alone or isolated because they are likely facing different issues than other people in their lives. Support groups offer a chance for people to come together and talk about common concerns, successes, and disappointments. Seeing how others cope with diabetes may give members of the group ideas for new ways of thinking about diabetes. Discussing strategies and experimenting with new information can open up a wealth of opportunities that helps participants become more knowledgeable about themselves and their diabetes. Sharing feelings and developing comrades through similar experiences can help patients feel less alone. Sometimes knowing that others are struggling with the same problems lifts some of the burden of having a chronic disease and gives patients the energy to meet yet another day with diabetes.

Offering patients the option by asking if a support group appeals to them is certainly appropriate. It is important to realize, however, that there are patients for whom support groups are not a desirable option. They may feel uncomfortable speaking in a group or find that the group adds stress to their lives by becoming one more obligation. Other strategies, such as an online support group, may help them to feel less alone. You could also help them identify a diabetes supporter in their life by creating a formal peer-counseling program or by linking patients who seem to hit it off in a group class. All of these options may create opportunities for interaction and decrease isolation.

46

My patients have told me that they want a support group, but I'm already doing an evening education program. How can I do a support group without taking more time from my family?

 Tip

Family relationships are just as important to diabetes educators as they are to our patients with diabetes. As an educator, you are not responsible to be all things to all patients. Although some diabetes education programs offer support groups, it is not always necessary for a diabetes educator to bear the sole responsibility for creating and running a support group. A peer-led support group may be the solution to your dilemma. Think of participants from past or present classes who might help organize and lead a support group and ask about their interest in doing so. If you have an advisory committee for your diabetes self-management education program, talking with the other members of the group, particularly the consumer member and a member with behavioral/psychosocial expertise, might help you identify potential leaders. A social worker or psychologist in your setting may be willing to train and supervise a peer leader. You could facilitate the initial planning meetings, serve as a resource, and market the group to participants in your education program.

Your state's department of health or social services may also have a self-help clearinghouse that is well versed in assisting individuals who wish to establish peer-led self-help groups.

What should I say when my patients ask me how to choose a support group?

 Tip

Not all support groups are created equal. This is a good thing! People have different needs, and support groups are only helpful if they meet the needs of those who attend. If you are fortunate enough to have more than one support group in your area, maintain a list of when and where they are held and the population they serve, for example, type 1 patients, men only, retired or older type 2 patients, children with type 2 diabetes, Spanish-speaking participants, etc.

Along with specific populations, support groups can also offer different formats. Someone newly diagnosed with diabetes may want a support group with an emphasis on providing information about diabetes management, whereas others may benefit from a peer-led group that discusses personal issues, day-to-day experiences with diabetes, and the lessons participants have learned by caring for themselves.

Even if the setting where you work has a support group, offering patients several choices may help them find the right fit. Including a list of available groups as a handout in your diabetes self-management education program gives the information to those who would not feel comfortable or don't know to ask. Asking for feedback from patients you refer to support groups will help you make more appropriate recommendations.

E Bonus

I'd like to create a support group. Where do I start?

 Tip

Here are some suggestions on how to start a group.

- Conduct a needs assessment by mail or phone among previous class participants to determine if they are interested in meeting as a group. Ask if they would prefer a group that focuses on education or support. Also poll patients for the location, time of day, and day of the week that would be most convenient and make sure this coincides with your availability and schedule.

- Obtain the support of your supervisor and any others in your setting as needed.

- Get help from others, including colleagues, your diabetes self-management education program advisory committee, and previous patients.

- Create a planning committee made up of those patients who expressed an interest in the group. If possible, include a social worker or psychologist on the committee. They will be a valuable addition, especially if group facilitation and psychosocial issues are not your strong suit.

- Develop a purpose or mission statement and define the goals for the program and strategies you will use to achieve them. Create benchmarks for the program to measure its effectiveness. Set a time to evaluate your support group to be sure that the needs of the participants are being met and that it is meeting its goals.

- Advertise the support group in your hospital newsletter, local or community newspapers, and with flyers or phone calls to past patients, especially those who participated in the needs assessment. Include the statement of purpose and a map. Your hospital public relations department may also be helpful in marketing your group.

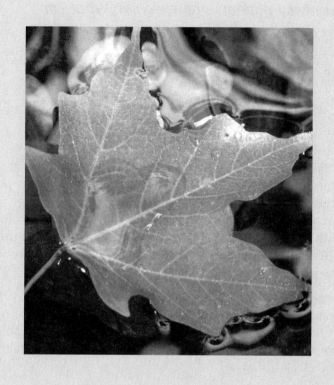

CHALLENGING

PATIENTS

48

***A** lot of my patients are in denial. What can I do to help them accept their diabetes?*

 Tip

Denial is a very common first reaction to bad news and also a protective mechanism that can actually be quite useful. If we are powerless to affect the outcome, denial protects us from spending energy worrying about a problem that we cannot change. It gives people time to allow the information to gradually become part of their thinking and their lives. Many patients with diabetes initially feel powerless and feel that the complications are inevitable.

However, denial that lasts is generally not useful in diabetes. Diabetes can be treated and its complications prevented. It can be very frustrating for health care providers when we see patients who refuse to believe that diabetes is serious or to do the things they need to do to take care of themselves.

As much as we would like to get through to these patients, we cannot force them to stop denying a problem. Often, attempts at confronting situations backfire. Denial is a response to fear, and confrontation usually increases fear. Patients often become more deeply steeped in their denial when confronted, and they consequently sometimes withdraw from care. What we can do as health professionals is express our concerns to patients. Such statements include, "I am concerned because of the decisions you are making to care for your diabetes. Based on what I have seen with other patients, I worry about what will happen. What do you think about your future with diabetes?" The purpose of this question is not to change the patient's denial, but rather to express your care and concern. It is a way of meeting your responsibility as a health care professional.

49

A lot of people I see seem overwhelmed with the diagnosis of diabetes and don't seem to listen when I start teaching them the survival skills they need. How can I get their attention?

 Tip

Sometimes coping is the first survival skill people with diabetes need to learn. Rather than beginning by teaching, spend a little time assessing where patients are emotionally. Although we all feel time pressures and it's easy to think that you are wasting your time, you are in reality wasting more time if you begin teaching before your patients are ready to learn.

Asking your patients what diabetes means to them is often a good place to start. Questions such as, "How did you feel?" or "What were your thoughts?" or "What went through your mind when you were diagnosed?" will help you establish a relationship with patients and help them view you as a source of support and information. A discussion about coping with diabetes may give them the first survival skill they need to learn.

50

Some of my patients feel helpless and hopeless. I find that I dread their visits because I am so drained by the end. How can I help them?

 Tip

People who feel hopeless and helpless can drain our energy if we spend our time trying to motivate or cheer them up. We can use up all of our energy trying to give some to them. These are also patients who never seem to get anywhere with their diabetes care and remain stuck on the same issues. These issues are usually presented as outside their control, such as, "My family won't drink low-fat milk."

How can we help patients to get unstuck? One strategy we can use is to confront the issue gently but assertively. For example, you may say, "I feel as though we discuss the same issues every time that you visit. I am concerned that we are not moving forward. Do you feel as if you are stuck?" Give these patients the opportunity to express their feelings of helplessness and hopelessness. Discuss the fact that no one can motivate them except themselves. Ask, "What will happen if things don't change?" and "Are you willing to accept that consequence?"

Sometimes you will agree that this is not the time for a particular patient to work on his or her diabetes care. Let the patient know that your door is open and that you will be available in the future. Help the patient to find other sources of support.

These are also patients whose visits take a long time because they are so needy. One approach is to begin the visit by saying, "We have 15 minutes to spend together today. How can I be of most help to you?"

Some patients who feel helpless and hopeless are clinically depressed. High blood glucose readings can also contribute to these feelings. It is important to screen all patients with diabetes for depression and offer referral to mental health workers as indicated.

51

A couple of my patients have said, "I made up all the numbers in my blood glucose log," as they handed me their logbook. I didn't know what to say. Any suggestions?

 Tip

Using a nonjudgmental tone, repeat their statement, "You made up your blood glucose? Help me understand why you felt you needed to make up your numbers." Give them time to respond. Their reasons may include fear of judgment, criticism, or blame by health care professionals or family members or a need for acceptance.

If patients tell you they made up their numbers, they are uncomfortable with what they did. The fact that they told you indicates that they trust you, and trust is the basic element of a therapeutic relationship. You might respond, "I am really glad you told me." You then need to assess what is going on with the patient by asking questions such as, "Is the regimen not working or too intense?" or "Have I conveyed that I am judging you based on your blood glucose levels?" Once you have an understanding of the patients and their needs, you can work with them to build on the trust they placed in you.

52

Some patients seem so demanding that they take a great deal of the team's time, yet we do not seem to get anywhere with them. Do you have any advice?

 Tip

Demanding patients and families can be very frustrating, especially when you don't seem to be moving toward a goal.

What is driving the demanding patient? Often issues of fear and anxiety make patients appear demanding when they are worried about their own health and safety. Listening carefully to their concerns and helping the patient and family identify their issues is a good starting place.

Patients are usually aware of what the issues are but may need help in clarifying problems so that they can create a plan. Try writing down a list of problems so they can see all of the issues they have identified. The patient may choose to pick one issue or problem on which to work. Helping patients identify strategies and a goal to work toward provides a framework for tackling problems. This makes problems less over-whelming and helps patients feel more in control of their lives. Engaging other members of the team provides a comprehensive plan and prevents a "splitting" of the team.

Communicating the plan to other members of the team is essential. It helps all team members reinforce the strategies and helps the patient and their family stay on course. When patients call or come in, all team members can work with the patient and revise the plan as needed.

53

I have had patients with major vision loss. How can I help them find needed resources?

 Tip

You can familiarize yourself with the lists of resources provided by your state health department. The American Diabetes Association's *Type 2 Diabetes: A Curriculum for Patients and Health Professionals* lists several resources in the support materials section and includes contact information. You can also look for additional listings on the ADA web site, www.diabetes.org, and the American Association of Diabetes Educators' web site, www.aadenet.org. Also, the magazine *Diabetes Forecast* publishes an annual resource guide issue. Finally, local organizations that assist the blind are also good sources of information.

If your patient is designated as legally blind, he or she may qualify to apply for special adaptive training. Some states have state-funded residential training centers that teach independent living. Many of these agencies will have information on laws to protect your patient and may highlight public facilities that have made provisions for those with visual impairments.

Inform your patient of the possibilities of devices that may sustain their independence. Other points to consider include the following:

- Contact meter companies to investigate which meters are more user-friendly for the visually impaired. For example, it is important to avoid confusion as to which button is for memory and which is for time and date.

- Downloadable meters may be useful so the patient/provider can plot values on a larger screen or in large print.

- Meters with auditory guides can be obtained with a prescription from many meter companies.

54

Some of my adult patients act like rebellious teenagers. They do things that they know will adversely affect their blood glucose in order to teach their physicians, family, or me "a lesson." How can I help them?

 Tip

If your patients are responding like teenagers, perhaps it is because they feel they are being treated like children. If they view diabetes self-management as others telling them what to do and making judgments about their behavior, they may respond as they did when they were teenagers. They may be disobedient (noncompliant) just to show you that they are in control of their lives.

The way to break this cycle is to step out of the parental role. Acknowledge that patients have the right and responsibility to decide how (and even if) they are going to manage their diabetes. Let patients know that you know it was common in the past for patients to be treated as naughty children. Let them know that you view patients as adults. The aim is to establish an adult relationship rather than one based on a parent–child paradigm.

Patients will likely test you. They will probably tell you all of the "bad" things that they have been doing. Responses such as, "Did that work for you?" or "What did you learn?" demonstrate that the judgment about these behaviors will be made by them and not by you. Once patients realize that they do not have to prove to themselves or others that they are in charge of their own lives, they can make self-management decisions based on the consequences rather than the need to show "who's the boss."

Some of my patients are "free spirits" and don't have any sort of routine. I find that their glucose swings are phenomenal. How can I help them?

 Tip

The world would be a dull place without a few free spirits! But determine if they are truly free spirits or acting out because of their diagnosis of diabetes.

Ask about their lifestyle and routine before they were diagnosed. If they were free spirits before they had diabetes, then working with them to design a highly flexible program is critical. This is particularly true for patients who take insulin and for whom safety is a concern.

Begin by letting them know the options for treatment that will provide them with the most flexibility. Point out that frequent testing and frequent shots can offer more flexibility but also greater responsibility and risks. Inquire about their experiences with hypoglycemia and ways that they can prevent its occurrence. Beginning statements with, "I am concerned about . . ." is more likely to get a positive response. After all, not even free spirits want to end up in the hospital or in an automobile accident.

After safety issues have been resolved, ask what other issues are problematic for these patients. Work with them to come up with self-management experiments they can do to find the least intrusive way to manage their diabetes. Conducting a series of collaboratively developed self-management experiments is likely to lead to a plan that represents a balance between freedom, safety, and diabetes care.

56

Some of my patients are working but have no health insurance or prescription drug coverage. How can I help them get the things they need to care for their diabetes?

 Tip

Many people are working part-time or are in jobs that do not provide health insurance. This seems to occur often among younger people, for whom the cost of supplies and medications for diabetes and other comorbidities can be staggering! Usually, the first step is to refer them to the social work department at your hospital to see if there are resources available.

Here are some other ideas on how to support your patients.

- Organizations such as the Salvation Army, Lion's Club, or local charities have programs that provide short-term financial assistance.

- Suggest that they ask their providers for medication samples or to prescribe generic versions of the drugs they are taking.

- Offer information about meters that use less expensive strips.

- Ask patients which blood glucose reading gives them the best information. Help patients to then develop a blood glucose testing plan that gives them the most information from the least number of tests.

- Inform patients of health fairs, free eye screenings, and blood pressure screenings in your area.

- Collect and make available coupons for strips or medications from pharmaceutical representatives or magazines.

Tip *Continued*

■ If you offer group classes or a support group, ask participants to call several area pharmacies and inquire about pricing for strips, syringes, and medication. Discuss their findings at the next meeting.

■ Most pharmaceutical and meter companies have assistance programs. Talk with the local representative or check out their web site. A list of these programs can be found at www.edhayes.com/indigentprogram.html.

57

My patients bring up a lot of problems, but when I suggest solutions, they come up with reasons why they won't work. I think of these as "yeah, but" patients. Can you offer any suggestions?

 Tip

When you talk about problems you are experiencing to your friends, do you want them to solve the problem or help you reflect on the issue and come up with your own solution? Most of the time we know that others can't solve the issue for us, we just need someone who can listen effectively. Most of us react with a "yeah, but" when other people tell us what to do, even if we don't say it.

Patients are the experts on their lives, and this includes their lives with diabetes. You can best serve your patients by helping them to solve their own problems. Activities such as the one below can be used in a group session or with an individual patient. In a group class, you can ask that patients do this independently or ask one member of the group to identify a problem he or she would like the rest of the group to help think about.

Ask the following questions:

- Being as specific as you can, what problem or barrier are you experiencing?
- How has this problem hindered or affected you?
- How does this problem make you feel?
- What do you gain if you keep this problem (e.g., able to fit in, don't want to change, don't feel I can make a change)?
- If you solve the problem, what do you gain?
- How have you dealt with problems in the past? What has worked and what hasn't?

57

Tip *Continued*

Next, ask the patients to list all of the options they can think of and identify the pluses and minuses of each potential solution. Suggest that they pick one they think has the best chance of working and ask if they want to experiment with this behavior.

If patients are truly stuck, statements such as, "This solution has worked for some of my patients. Do you think it would work for you?" or "Would it help for me to make some suggestions from which you can choose?" offer options but still give the responsibility for solving problems to the patient.

Self-selected solutions are the most meaningful and are as personal and varied as the number of patients you see. When it comes to problems, the questions need to come from you and the answers from the patient.

F Bonus

__M__any of my patients have financial needs that I cannot meet, but I want to be helpful. Do you have any suggestions?

 Tip

Patients often have multiple needs, many of which you won't be able to meet. Luckily, there are usually a variety of resources available in your hospital and community. If you think that you have to provide information about all of a patient's needs, you will feel overwhelmed, especially if you are in the early phase of your work as a diabetes educator. Think about your typical patient and the type of resources your patients need most often. If you have a social work department in your facility, meeting with the staff and describing your target population might be a good place to begin. Listings of available resources are often available from community or state health departments and local diabetes organizations.

Specific options can include the following:

■ Financial help is often available through referral to the social work department in your facility, the auxiliary or volunteer organization in your hospital, local churches, and charitable organizations such as the Lion's club, Salvation Army, and others.

■ Scholarships to your education program can be solicited from private individuals, local businesses, and pharmaceutical and durable medical equipment companies in return for advertising.

■ The social work department and community mental health clinics can help with family counseling and other psychological services.

■ Meals-on-Wheels, home care, and other elderly support services can help patients remain independent.

■ There are resources designed for patients with special needs, for example, children or patients with complications from diabetes. The Internet, the yellow pages, or the community health department in your state often list these resources.

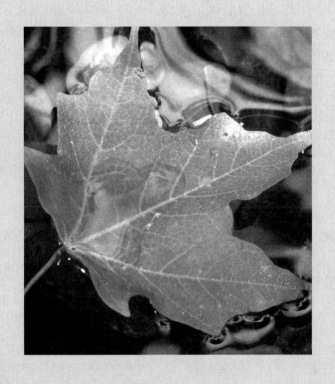

EATING AND

PHYSICAL

ACTIVITY

58

I know that many of my patients would benefit from exercise, but they often seem to get turned off when I bring up the subject. Do you have any suggestions?

 Tip

Part of the problem may be the word "exercise." The words "exercise" and "diet" have taken on such negative connotations that in most instances, we would be better off not using those words at all. Many patients have developed negative associations with these words based on their experiences trying to follow a rigid diet or maintain an exercise regimen, e.g., 30 minutes a day on a treadmill. Even if we are talking about a gradual and incremental approach to physical activity, many patients tune out if we use the word "exercise."

It may be more helpful to talk with patients about the amount of physical activity that they engage in over the course of a normal day. You can then discuss current research, which indicates that increases in activities such as walking or climbing stairs, even if done in short increments (e.g., three times a day for 10 minutes), can contribute to improved cardiovascular health and blood glucose control. This is more appealing for many patients, particularly those who have been very sedentary for some time.

59

I can understand why the term "physical activity" is generally preferable to the word "exercise," but how can I help patients choose a physical activity program?

 Tip

When patients express a particular interest in beginning a defined exercise program such as jogging or aerobic dancing, we help them get started. However, many patients do not have much long-term success with such structured exercise programs. If, after patients consider the costs and benefits of becoming more active, they express an interest in physical activity, we suggest that they look for opportunities to increase physical activity during the course of a day. For example, they might decide to park farther away from their workplace each morning, which will add two-, five-, or ten-minute walks to each workday. A patient who works on the tenth floor of a building and usually takes the elevator might decide to walk up one or two flights of stairs and then take the elevator. Over time, that patient might increase the number of floors he or she reaches by climbing the stairs.

As one of our mentors summarized, "It's easier to ride a horse in the direction it's going." Changes in activities that people engage in routinely are usually easier to make and sustain than the more substantial changes involved in adding a structured exercise program such as jogging or swimming. We have one patient who parks on the lowest level of the parking garage each morning and walks up all the ramps to the top level where there is an overpass that goes into the building where he works. He reports that this activity is easy to maintain because it has become such a habit.

60

Some of my patients say, "Just tell me what to eat." They expect a written diet or meal plan that will help them to control their diabetes. What advice do you have about helping patients consider a flexible approach to meal planning?

 Tip

It's not surprising that some patients take this approach to meal planning because it was a standard practice for many years for physicians and other health professionals to simply prescribe an ADA diet. The myth of an "ADA diet" persists to this day even though only a small number of patients were ever able to use one effectively.

If your patients want a standard meal plan, give them one. Suggest that they experiment with the plan for a couple of weeks and see how it fits into their lives. A follow-up visit or phone call is essential to discuss the results of the experiment and to evaluate the benefits and limitations of the meal plan. After a few weeks of trying to use a standard diet, many patients become motivated to learn how to change the meal plan to better fit their preferences and circumstances.

61

I have a number of patients who say they feel guilty when they "cheat" on their meal plan. How can I help them not to think of it as cheating?

 Tip

Cheating is a term that reflects guilt for doing what we believe is the wrong thing, when we think no one is looking. It often involves taking an unfair advantage at the expense of another person. In the case of a meal plan, there is no other person who is cheated and the expense is only incurred by the patient.

Patients may choose the word "cheat" in their effort to accept responsibility and to maintain our approval. Some patients are very hard on themselves for not following the routine but seldom sort out the reasons why they "cheated." But in fact, saying they cheated is really a way to skirt responsibility. In reality, they make a choice that is both their right and their responsibility.

One response is to ask whom did they cheat? Often the response is, "I knew the right thing to do, and I didn't do it." Ask them why. Questions to help them better evaluate their decision are: "What were the circumstances surrounding your choice? What was the consequence? Was it worth it? What did you learn from the experience? What would you do differently next time?"

It is essential that we remain neutral and nonjudgmental and ask questions that help patients achieve clarity for themselves.

62

__H__ow can I help patients who tell me that they never eat certain foods because they can't stop eating once they start?

 Tip

Patients identifying problem foods may feel they lack control over this food. Avoiding the food may cause them to feel deprived and result in bingeing. There are several questions that can help patients clarify their fears and identify patterns.

What makes the food a problem? If they feel very hungry—possibly on days when they have only eaten one meal—do they feel more susceptible to bingeing on this food? Do they eat this food when they are lonely, angry, bored, or experiencing some other negative emotion?

If patients identify problem foods, ask them, "Is that the only food you eat in excess?" If the patient feels deprived, a strategy to incorporate the food in moderation might help. For example, what if the food was planned as part of a meal? Could they imagine that after eating that meal, they would continue to eat excess amounts? The answers to these questions will help focus the discussion on the particulars of this patient's problem.

If they believe that eating a particular food will cause their blood sugars to go way up, suggest an experiment to try the food with a meal and then test their blood glucose two hours later to see if the negative consequence they fear occurs. Other strategies include purchasing foods in single-serving containers or pre-portioning foods. Others may need to talk about the meaning that problem foods have for them, such as emotional attachments to family traditions or associations with pleasant memories. Sometimes just recognizing the emotional attachment to food is sufficient. It is often useful for patients to acknowledge that they are responding to stress or other emotions when they binge. Others may benefit from referral to a mental health worker.

63

Some patients who are referred to me are overwhelmed by the changes they have been told to make in their diets. Can I do anything to help ease this process for them?

 Tip

The first step is to explore with your patients the feelings of being overwhelmed. As they express why they are overwhelmed, you will gain important insights and clues to reactions based on dietary recommendations that may well be inappropriate and/or out-of-date. The second step is to assess what the patients want. The third step is to reassure patients that dietary changes can be made using small and progressive steps that can help them achieve their goals. Once patients understand that modest changes in the way they eat can have a positive impact on their health, they may wish to consider taking the first step. At subsequent visits, we discuss what helped or hindered their progress. We ask our patients if they are willing to try more steps and encourage them to share their experiences with us, that is, we ask them what they are learning about what does and doesn't work for them as they pursue their goals.

64

I have several patients who say that, "Eating is no fun any more since I developed diabetes." How can I help them?

 Tip

Eating for many patients becomes a chore as they lose some of the spontaneity that they had before they got diabetes. Counting carbs, reading labels, making choices, eating new or different foods, and monitoring blood glucose after meals can become burdensome. Balancing the pleasure of food today with the risks of complications can also reduce the enjoyment of meals.

Ask patients to identify what was fun about eating before they had diabetes and what would help make it fun again. These questions may help you find that patients have unnecessarily restricted favorite foods and can be more flexible in their meal choices. You may find out that their family sets the rules for their food choices. You may find out that they don't like to weigh or measure. Once you find problems, work with the patient to develop ideas to make eating easier and fun again.

65

I have patients who are being treated for an eating disorder. What can I do to support their efforts?

 Tip

Your support as an educator is valuable. Although it is usually better not to ask such patients about weight changes or comment on their appearance, expressing your concern and offering your support is helpful. Express your willingness to listen—and avoid offering advice.

If you do help your patients plan meals to manage their blood glucose levels, you can help them evaluate their food selections using blood glucose monitoring.

During recovery, your patients may struggle with real versus perceived consequences of certain behaviors. One strategy is to ask patients to write their troubling thoughts. Typically, the thoughts or assertions are magnified, for example, "Because I am eating this I will be big as a house," or "I have already blown it today so I may as well eat it all." Discussing real consequences versus the ones the patient has imagined is useful. An example of real consequences would be, "Yes, my blood glucose will go up, but I can help myself by . . ." Support your patient's decision to get treatment and encourage him or her to stick with it.

66

Are there clues that could alert me to the possibility that some of my patients have eating disorders such as anorexia, bulimia, or compulsive eating?

 Tip

Patients with low self-esteem and/or a negative body image are at higher risk for eating disorders. Clues are patients who may

- severely restrict fats, calories, or pleasurable foods
- consume excessive amounts of diet beverages or diet foods
- have a fear of getting fat or have strong perceptions of most foods as harmful or fattening
- experience tremendous guilt after eating normal to large portions of foods
- complain of feeling out of control when eating large portions of foods
- cycle through multiple fad diets
- manipulate insulin dosages inappropriately (e.g., "spilling glucose," usually to lose weight)
- induce vomiting, use laxatives or diuretics, and/or exercise excessively
- complain of constipation, loss of menses (in women who are premenopausal), low blood pressure, dizziness or headaches, loss of hair, or swollen neck glands

The presence of these clues indicates a need to further assess the presence of an eating disorder. Some patients may readily admit that they are dealing with an eating disorder, whereas others may not realize that their behavior is symptomatic of an eating disorder. One or more of these clues indicate that you may need to refer the patient to another health professional with expertise in eating disorders.

Tip *Continued*

Here are a few resources that will help you to learn more about the diagnosis of an eating disorder and how to help:

- www.edap.org
- www.something-fishy.org
- www.eatingdisorders.mentalhelp.net
- www.anred.com

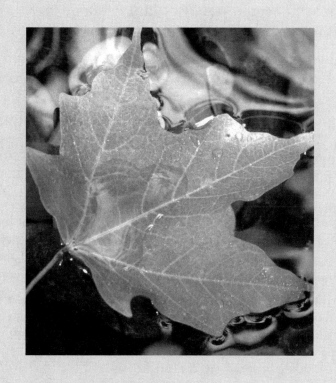

EDUCATOR–PATIENT

RELATIONSHIPS

67

How can I keep a positive attitude about my patients?

 Tip

Getting to know your patients as people is a good start. What is important to them? What do they like to do for fun? What do you know about their family?

Building a meaningful relationship with your patients helps you see all aspects of their lives. This helps you understand how diabetes affects their daily lives and allows you to see them as more than a "diabetic." This also helps you celebrate the successes and understand the disappointments they have.

As educators, we often act as cheerleaders for our patients and families. The day-to-day care that diabetes requires is fatiguing for patients and their families. As educators, we have the privilege of being involved in a very personal aspect of our patients' lives. Our nonjudgmental caring and understanding is very powerful medicine.

68

I've heard the phrase "taking the walk with your patients." What does this mean?

 Tip

Taking the walk with your patient means creating a partnership. When you walk with a patient, you respect his or her right to make decisions and refrain from making judgments about his or her choices. At the same time, the patient understands the need to accept responsibility for his or her own care and choices.

Because taking the walk with the patient is different than traditional care where health professionals serve as leaders, patients often don't understand the need to work collaboratively with their caregivers. The first step of walking with patients is to tell them what your role is and what theirs will be. An effective approach is to begin the first interaction with patients or the first session of a class by letting them know that diabetes care is different. We also acknowledge that we are not experts on their lives or on what diabetes means to them. We then point out that they need to become equal partners. We tell patients that we want to take the walk *with* them but that we cannot take it *for* them. We are here to facilitate, inform, support, and inspire.

Diabetes is a journey, and health professionals and patients can be traveling companions once they recognize the importance of a partnership.

69

I have been learning a lot about patient-centered care lately. What are some things I can do to put patients at the center of our care?

 Tip

One important way is to create a patient-centered environment. This type of environment shows patients that we value and care for and about them. We demonstrate that we put patients first when confidentiality and privacy are respected, waiting time is minimized, the patient's agenda for each visit is addressed, and the physical environment is as pleasant as possible.

Patient-centered visits are a critical part of this type of approach. When you enter the room and greet your patients by saying, "How are you?" do they respond by telling you about issues or concerns or by handing you their blood glucose logbook? Because so much of diabetes care is focused on adjusting therapy to manage blood glucose levels, we may inadvertently send patients the message that we are more interested in their numbers than in them. We have found that asking patients at the start of a visit to identify the areas that they would like addressed has changed our practice in a positive way. The visit becomes far more satisfying because communication is enhanced. The time is spent more efficiently because we are working towards a common goal for that visit. It also eliminates the patient saying, "Oh, just one more thing . . ." as we walk out the door. That "one thing" is sometimes a serious problem that takes longer to deal with than the initial part of the visit. Getting that problem on the table early is far more efficient.

Useful phrases for initiating a patient-centered visit or educational session include the following:

■ What issues about your diabetes would you like to work on or talk about today?

Tip *Continued*

■ How do you think things are going with your diabetes?

■ What concerns you most about your diabetes?

■ What would you like to address or accomplish before you leave here today?

■ What is the hardest thing for you about your diabetes?

70

I have had patients tell me that I don't know what it's like to have diabetes. How can I respond?

 Tip

A good place to begin is by acknowledging that the statement is correct. Let patients know that you don't know what it is like with a statement such as, "You're right, I don't know." Each person's experience is unique in many respects. Even educators with diabetes can't know for sure how another person experiences diabetes. For one person, having diabetes may seem like a disaster, whereas for another person, it may seem like a challenge.

Ask patients to describe their experience with diabetes. Questions such as, "Tell me what having diabetes is like for you," or "What does having diabetes mean to you?" are responsive to the issue raised. By asking these questions, you may encourage patients to really think about their diagnosis and how it fits into their lives—perhaps for the first time. Both you and the patients will gain a better understanding of their experience with diabetes.

I *have heard that it is more effective to ask patients to identify strategies to solve their own problems rather than to tell them what I think they need to do. Will they think that I don't know what I'm doing?*

 Tip

Have you ever told a problem to a friend and had them say, "Here's what you should do"? How do you respond? Most of us smile, nod, and silently decide to ignore their advice and to choose another friend with whom to discuss our problems. Our patients come to us to get skills and information so that they can manage their diabetes. Diabetes care is our area of expertise. But solving our patients' problems requires another area of expertise that we don't have. We are not experts on our patients' lives. That is their area of expertise.

When you attempt to solve patients' problems, one of several things may happen. The solution you suggest may

- help resolve the problem
- not be tried because the patient doesn't believe the option will work
- work for a short time only
- not work for that particular patient even though other patients have found it effective

Although the solutions we suggest work occasionally, often they do not. When our solutions don't work, we can look incompetent. Our patients may decide that we don't know what we are talking about when our solutions don't work out for them.

Solutions that are self-identified are self-motivating. When we help our patients to identify their own solutions and use the problem-solving process, we convey our respect and our competence.

72

Other than telling patients my philosophy of diabetes self-management, are there other ways that I can convey it to them?

 Tip

Although we can use words to describe our philosophy, the words that we use every day when we talk about diabetes self-management will often more powerfully reveal and communicate our true vision. When we speak, we communicate much more than the literal meaning of the words. Think about the phrases that you use while teaching and what they convey. Statements such as, "You should check your feet every day," or "Your doctor wants your A1C in the normal range," or "We like for our patients to check their blood glucose at least three times a day," convey a more traditional approach to education. The patient is asked to perform self-care for the purpose of pleasing the health professional or because these are the diabetes self-management "rules" that patients are expected to follow.

Statements such as, "Because you have these three numb areas on your feet, checking these places every day can help you find a problem before it becomes serious," or "An A1C closer to normal has been shown to reduce your risks for complications," are designed to help patients make an informed decision rather than simply comply with the treatment plan.

Written materials also convey a tone that reflects the author's philosophy. It is often helpful to read materials you use and pretend that you are a patient hearing the words for the first time. Do you feel informed, respected, and supported, or do you feel like a child who is being told what to do without being told why?

Although it's true that actions speak louder than words, the words that we choose speak more loudly than we think.

73

How can I make sure that my patients know I really care about them?

 Tip

There are many ways to convey caring to patients. We each have somewhat different ways of expressing how we feel. A few of the ways to express caring are listed below. Use those that feel most natural and comfortable for you.

- One of the most common ways of conveying caring is by touching. A light hand on the shoulder, a hug, or gently touching the hand of a patient who is upset all convey caring and concern. Nonverbal ways of expressing caring are often more potent than words. However, the decision to touch a patient requires using judgment about how the patient is likely to perceive being touched. Our facial expression, our posture (e.g., leaning toward the patient while sitting), eye contact, and paying complete attention to what our patients are saying are also ways that we can demonstrate caring.

- Another way is to begin every visit with a patient with one or two questions about the patient as a person (e.g., "How is your family?" or "How are things at work?"). One educator we know keeps a tickler file so that she can send a birthday card to each of her long-term patients.

- Educators can demonstrate caring through the character of the physical environment in which they interact with their patients. For example, plants, soft lighting, and artwork all tend to humanize what might be perceived as a clinical and impersonal environment. Having a dish of sugarless candies available or hanging posters on the wall that express humanistic values are ways of communicating to our patients that we care about them.

The secret is finding ways of expression that feel genuine and natural to you.

74

I have a few patients who just seem to rub me the wrong way. I'm less patient, empathetic, and effective with them. Do you have any ideas about what I can do?

 Tip

There are some people in the world who, given their individual personalities, tend to rub each other the wrong way. Given the unlikelihood that you are going to change either your personality or the patient's, you will probably have to decide whether you are able to provide such a patient with the care he or she needs and deserves. If you are not able to give your best to such a patient, it is appropriate to refer him or her to someone else.

However, this decision should only be made after some reflection. It may be useful to discuss a "difficult" patient and your reaction to that patient with a colleague that you trust and respect to get a different perspective. If you conclude that in fact the problem is "bad chemistry," the next step is to discuss the issue with the patient. This discussion will probably be a bit uncomfortable for both of you. You could begin by saying that you are concerned because you perceive your personality differences are interfering with your ability to provide the level of care that he or she deserves. You could ask the patient if he or she has had similar feelings of frustration or has felt disconnected from you. If after such a discussion the two of you conclude that a referral is in order, then you should facilitate this referral personally. The process will occur more smoothly if you have already discussed the patient with one of your colleagues and he or she has agreed to work with that patient.

There are a couple of important concerns if this referral process is to succeed. First, such patients must genuinely feel that they are being referred in order to ensure that they receive the best diabetes care and education. Second, your colleague must believe that you are not "dumping" your most difficult patients on him or her. If these concerns are addressed adequately, it is very likely that both you and the patient with whom you have "bad chemistry" will benefit from this change.

Some patients call frequently and want to talk about all their personal problems. Solving such problems isn't my job. What can I do?

 Tip

Try directing the conversation back to diabetes by asking, "How is this problem affecting your diabetes self-management?" If it becomes clear that the patient doesn't want to work on diabetes care, then the discussion is not an appropriate use of the diabetes educator's phone time. There are some things that we cannot do on the phone. Providing ongoing therapy and problem-solving for our patient's personal problems on the telephone can be an enabling behavior. We can actually get caught in a vicious circle of enabling patients and making them dependent on us. If our patients are calling frequently for emotional support and the phone calls are lengthy, we need to refer them to the appropriate resources for help. We can help them realize what their needs are and what the best resources are to help them.

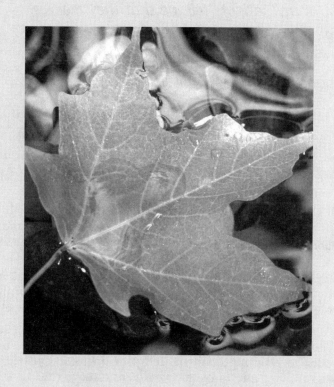

HELP FROM

OTHER HEALTH

PROFESSIONALS

75

A lot of my patients tell me that they feel intimidated when they visit their doctor. What can I do to help them create a collaborative relationship with their physician?

 Tip

It can be intimidating for many of us to see our physicians. The situation can make even the most assertive person feel like a child. Here are several tips that will help your patients feel less intimidated and create a more collaborative relationship.

- Have organized and ready any specific information that you think your provider will want. Prepare for your appointment the way that you would prepare for a work meeting or other type of assignment.

- Write down any questions that you would like to ask, and take the list to your appointment. Tell your doctor at the beginning that you have questions that you want to have time to ask before the end of the visit.

- Bring in any web site or newspaper stories to show your physician. Don't rely on your memory regarding the source.

- Set your own agenda for the appointment. Think ahead about what you want to leave knowing and doing. Short visits can be effective if they are focused.

- Set and know your own goals for your health, and talk about them with your doctor. Ask your doctor if those are reasonable goals for you or if your physician has a different opinion. You can use that information to help you make an informed decision.

76

A lot of my patients tell me they leave their doctor's appointment frustrated because they don't feel that their needs were met. What can I do to help them get more out of their appointments?

 Tip

There are several tips that will help your patients get the most out of their appointments.

- Tell your doctor at the start of the appointment if there are specific concerns or questions that you want to have addressed at the visit. Don't wait to be asked—speak up.

- Keep track of annual and other tests of your diabetes and its complications. Remind your doctor that you need a referral when it's time for follow-up visits.

- When your doctor orders tests, ask about their purpose and the reason that the test was ordered at this time. Actively seek out the results and ask what they mean.

- Be honest with your doctor. If you are having trouble with your diabetes self-care, tell your doctor why. You can use the opportunity to problem-solve and look for solutions together.

- Speak up if your doctor is not meeting your needs. Although it can be uncomfortable, the result may be life-saving or life-changing care.

77

Do you have any advice about when to refer patients to a mental health professional for psychosocial issues?

 Tip

There are three situations in which a referral to a psychologist or social worker may be indicated. The first is if the patient wants such a referral. This is not to suggest we have to wait until the patient asks to be referred, but rather there may be times when it would be wise to say, "Would you like to talk to a psychologist or counselor about this issue?" If the patient says "yes," then a referral is indicated. The second indication is when, as an educator, you feel like you are in over your head regarding a psychosocial problem. This is a somewhat subjective indicator because it will vary among educators, but if you are clearly uncomfortable pursuing a psychosocial issue introduced by a patient, then it is time to refer. The third criterion is when the psychosocial aspect of diabetes has become a significant problem in its own right and is undermining the ability of the patient to function effectively either psychologically or in the area of diabetes self-management. For example, a patient who wishes to talk about the frustrations of having been diagnosed with diabetes and needing to make major lifestyle changes may not need a referral, as long as these feelings are not immobilizing him or her. However, a referral is clearly indicated for patients whose anxiety or depression is undermining their ability to function effectively and enjoy life. Because rates of depression are significantly higher for patients with diabetes than for the general population, this is an important problem to look for. Given the fact there are many effective cognitive and pharmaceutical treatments for depression, referral at the earliest indication of this condition is generally a good idea.

78

Some of my patients seem pretty anxious about having diabetes. How do I decide whether to refer them to a mental health professional for this problem?

 Tip

Anxiety, like many psychological experiences, is a continuum that goes from no anxiety at all to absolutely paralyzing anxiety. A moderate amount of anxiety is a natural and appropriate reaction to having a chronic disease such as diabetes. In fact, anxiety is part of what motivates most patients to seek out diabetes education and to make a serious effort at diabetes self-management. However, if our patients' anxiety level is too high, it will interfere with their ability to learn and manage their illness. Strong anxiety can also interfere with other parts of their lives, such as eating, sleeping, and relationships. It can significantly detract from the quality of their lives.

The best way to determine a patient's level of anxiety is to discuss it with him or her. For example, you can ask patients if their diabetes makes them feel anxious. If patients report that their level of anxiety significantly interferes with their diabetes self-management, ability to learn, ability to function normally, and/or quality of life, then it would be appropriate to suggest that they seek a formal evaluation from a qualified mental health professional. Remind overly anxious patients that there are effective treatments for anxiety and that they do not have to suffer unnecessarily. If patients report trying to learn about diabetes and seek the best medical care to lessen their anxiety, then their level is probably appropriate to the challenges they are facing.

Bottom line: if you are at all uncertain about whether the patient's level of anxiety warrants professional help, err on the side of safety and refer the patient for an evaluation.

H Bonus

Many of my patients seem depressed. How can I find out if I need to refer them for counseling?

 Tip

Clinical depression is a serious problem that occurs twice as often among people with diabetes. It has a negative effect on both quality of life and diabetes management. Research has shown that depression is significantly linked with mortality among patients with diabetes. Unless you are a psychologist, social worker, mental health nurse specialist, or psychiatrist, you cannot do a full assessment of clinical depression. However, you can screen* for depression among your patients by asking the below questions.

In the past year:

- Have you had two weeks or more during which you felt sad, blue, or depressed most of the time?
- Have you had two weeks or more during which you lost all interest or pleasure in things that you normally cared about or enjoyed?
- Have you lost or gained a lot of weight?
- Are you eating more or less than usual?
- Have you had trouble sleeping, or are you sleeping too much?
- Have you had trouble making decisions or focusing on things?

Also ask the patient, "Have you had two or more years in your life when you felt sad or blue most days, even if you felt okay sometimes? If yes, have you felt depressed or sad much of the time in the past year?"

Answering "yes" to any of these questions means that additional assessment either through referral or by a qualified mental health professional in your program is needed.

*Reference for screening tool: www.mentalhealth.com

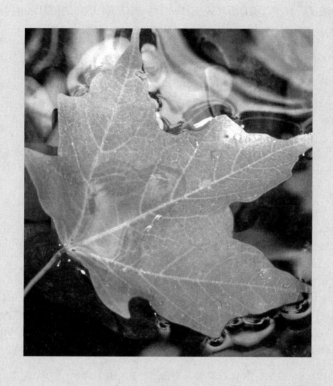

EDUCATOR

CONCERNS

79

Some of my patients have so many problems that we are both overwhelmed. How can I help them make the first step toward effective diabetes self-management?

 Tip

Diabetes on top of life's other problems overwhelms many patients. If you feel as though you are responsible for solving your patients' problems, it can also be overwhelming for you as an educator.

One strategy for an individual session is to keep track of the issues patients raise as they talk. Summarize the list, and then ask the patient to prioritize the issues. For example, you might say "I heard you describe four issues: your daughter's problems in school, the lack of support you feel from your spouse in dealing with her teacher, the fact that the stress has affected your blood glucose, and your tendency to overeat because of all of the tension. Are these the issues? Is there one on which you would like to focus today?"

In a group session, you can ask the group to list various problems that people with diabetes commonly encounter, or you can ask one person to tell about a problem he or she would like the group to work on. If your group is large, you can break up into smaller groups and have each group come up with several ideas for ways to deal with the problem, asking them to be as creative as they can. When you reconvene the larger group, have each of the smaller groups briefly describe the solutions. This type of activity helps you to integrate content with the practical and psychosocial aspects of diabetes care. For example, you can talk about the benefits of tight glucose control and then ask patients to propose solutions to the problems that tight control poses when implementing intensive management.

80

So many of my patients with type 2 diabetes seem unable or unwilling to make changes that I am beginning to feel burned out. Any suggestions?

 Tip

It is not surprising that you feel burned out if you are trying to do the impossible, that is, accept responsibility for changing another person's behavior. Burnout comes from seemingly unresolvable frustrations. This issue is resolved only when and if we truly recognize that we are not able to change or responsible for changing the behavior of our patients.

Simply agreeing with the above assertion is seldom enough to dissipate the frustration. Usually, true resolution only comes from seeing the impossibility of "being responsible for getting patients to change" in our actual experience with patients. The experiential recognition that we can't control our patients (and are therefore not responsible for their behavior) results in a kind of psychological letting go, where we stop trying to do the impossible. Failing to let go almost inevitably results in decreasing feelings of affinity for our patients and a diminishing sense of satisfaction with our work. Letting go of the tension arising from the effort to "get" patients to change can reenergize us and our work. It can allow us to reestablish caring relationships with our patients because our relationships will be based on realistic expectations and possibilities.

81

When one of my favorite patients died, I felt like I lost a good friend. I am having a hard time relating to some of my other patients now. How can I handle this?

 Tip

It is natural to care about our patients. The loss we feel when a patient with whom we have had a special relationship dies is appropriate and needs to be acknowledged. Talking with coworkers and sharing feelings and anecdotes about that person may help. Sending a sympathy card, writing a personal note mentioning the special connection you felt with the patient, calling a member of the family, making a donation in his or her name, or going to the funeral can be helpful for the family and for you. Sometimes we pull away from situations such as these because it seems as if there is nothing we can do that will make things better. Don't worry that you don't know what to say. There is nothing you can say that will change the situation. Expressing our sympathy to the patient's loved ones can help them and us move through the grieving process. It will probably be comforting for your patient's family and friends to know how their loved one touched your life and that you care.

Feeling a connection with the patients with whom we work is one of the benefits of being a diabetes educator. Our greatest professional joys often come from the relationships we create with the patients. Professionals can be professional and still allow themselves to feel loss. Not grieving or acknowledging feelings can increase burnout or cause you to pull away from patients you encounter in the future. Death is a part of life. Sadly, all too often, it comes early to those with diabetes.

82

My patients call me with reports about new advances in diabetes care they have seen on television or heard on the radio. I have heard some of these stories, but not all. How can I track down the real information?

 Tip

Many media reports concerning new advances in diabetes medications or products are from articles published in scientific journals. Sometimes these advances are still in the most basic phase of testing. "No more insulin shots for diabetes" could be a newspaper story headline referring to research that hasn't even progressed past animal testing. The media reports can make it sound as if new medication or technologies are available to consumers today when, in truth, they may be years away or may never happen.

Explain to patients that it takes most medications and durable medical goods between seven and ten years to come to market. A news report can occur at any point in this process. To find out information about a specific product, you can reference the U.S. Food and Drug Administration's web site (www.fda.gov), where recent product approvals are posted. You can also ask the patient to tell you the source of the report and contact the television/radio station or publication yourself. Most media outlets have a health reporter with whom you can speak about the story or the original article. If appropriate, you can also offer to clear up any misconceptions the reporter has about the story.

83

I get really upset when I'm out in public and overhear people saying things about diabetes that are wrong. Last week in a restaurant I heard someone say that people with diabetes should never have sugar. Should I say something to set the record straight?

 Tip

That's up to you—you may get some strange looks! Your decision to speak up or stay quiet may depend on the situation and the potential for patients being harmed or offended.

One option is to offer to speak to civic or other community-based organizations that frequently encounter people who have diabetes. Examples are senior citizen organizations, the Lion's Club, veterans groups, faith-based groups, or emergency medical services. Your expertise may be particularly helpful for groups who frequently serve food to a number of people with diabetes and want to be sure that it is appropriate for them.

The incidence of diabetes is on the rise and has received a great deal of media coverage. Many organizations appreciate a speaker who can give them an overview of diabetes. An effective way to begin your presentation to this type of group is with a true/false test of diabetes myths. This gives you opportunities to dispel many of the myths of diabetes and provides a way to reach the general public with new information about diabetes.

I thought that because I have diabetes I could really be empathetic to my patients. But I get really scared when I see patients with severe complications—especially if they have taken care of themselves. What can I do?

 Tip

Choosing diabetes education as a career when you have diabetes has benefits and costs. On the one hand, you can understand in a very real way much of what your patients go through every day. You also have colleagues who understand diabetes and can be supportive. On the other hand, you live with your diabetes 24 hours a day. Add working with patients who have diabetes eight to ten hours a day, and you are at risk for diabetes overload. Keep in mind that you are seeing a particular subset of the population of people with diabetes, so it is likely that some of your patients will experience complications. If you work in a specialty setting, you are probably seeing people with the most severe problems.

When you have diabetes and work as an educator, you may feel obligated to be a perfect patient. Imposing these expectations on yourself increases the likelihood that you will feel overwhelmed. You may also feel that because you have a chronic illness, you need to be superman or superwoman. You may need to remind yourself that it is okay to take a day off when you are feeling particularly overwhelmed or to ask another diabetes educator to see a patient who is particularly upsetting for you.

You may find that it helps to do a fun project related to diabetes, such as a walk or camp. Involvement with your local educators group can be supportive for you professionally and personally. If volunteering is draining for you, limit your involvement with diabetes outside of your work time. Diabetes doesn't need to be the only focus in your life, and you will likely be healthier if it isn't.

84

Tip *Continued*

If this is an ongoing concern, you may want to talk with a trusted colleague, a counselor, or your doctor. If your job is causing you a considerable amount of stress, you may need to consider leaving the field of diabetes education. Stress adds to the daily and long-term difficulties of managing diabetes. Although we need dedicated, caring diabetes educators, having a career that is detrimental to your health is not worth it.

85

I seem to have a lot of difficulty getting off the phone when talking with patients. Do you have any suggestions?

 Tip

Many practices have attempted to contain the phone time to "call-in hours," when care providers are available to handle urgent calls as they come in. The times are often set up first thing in the morning from 7:00 a.m. to 9:00 a.m. or from 8:00 a.m. to 10:00 a.m. and again at the end of the day from 3:00 p.m. to 5:00 p.m. Urgent calls are handled throughout the day as needed. Letting patients know how much time you have when you begin your call can help. Ask, "How can we best spend this time?" or suggest, "Let's focus on your primary concern." Also set clear guidelines for the calls.

Having a consistent way of handling calls among providers in the office is important. Patients can be confused if one person is willing to talk on the phone at length and the next provider is focused, helps create a plan, and gets off the phone quickly. Having patients and families fax or e-mail their blood glucose readings and questions can save a great deal of time. All the data are there for you. You can call or fax your suggestions. Some educators like having the patient and family e-mail information to them and to also respond by e-mail or phone. Patients and families who need lots of help on the phone may need to come in for a face-to-face visit and/or have their diabetes self-management education reevaluated.

86

How do I get my team of professionals to act like a real team?

 Tip

Creating an effective team takes commitment from all team members. The commitment involves time and valuing differing areas of expertise. One member needs to take the lead for bringing the group together and leading the meetings. Some strategies for creating a team include

- creating a common goal or mission statement (to keep you focused)
- meeting weekly to discuss issues (to keep you connected)
- seeking input from each team member (to affirm the importance of all members)
- committing to work through difficult team issues together (to create a bond through successful problem-solving)
- having fun together—knowing each team member on a personal basis enhances the commitment of the group

Consistency, continuity, and leadership are essential to keep the team on track. Group continuity is important because teams need time to develop the relationships necessary to become a whole that is more than the sum of its members. If team members are constantly changing, you don't have a team. Also, having the team meetings led by a facilitator who has good interpersonal skills is very important.

A consistent philosophy of care among a team of providers helps patients feel confident and secure.

87

I am so busy. What can I do to relieve stress?

 Tip

Knowing what causes you stress is the key. Feeling overwhelmed with your work and the many other competing demands in life can cause stress. Organizing work and the other aspects of your life can help you feel in control and decrease your sense of urgency and stress.

Sometimes we stay busy to avoid a situation we don't want to face, for example, a serious relationship problem. Ask yourself, "Is my 'busyness' a way of avoiding something?" If it is, then keeping busy will only make the stress worse by postponing facing a situation that is unlikely to solve itself.

You cannot prevent stress. Learning to cope with stressful events makes life easier. Exercising, meditating, going for a walk, and getting a massage are ways that help people handle stress.

Identify what you like to do, and take some time every day to do the things you like. These can be things that "renew" and reenergize you and can take very little time: having a cappuccino on the way to work, going for a walk at lunch, listening to music while working on the computer, taking some brief quiet time to reflect on your day before leaving the office, having lunch with a friend, laughing at your own mistakes, or working out. To care for others, we have to take care of ourselves.

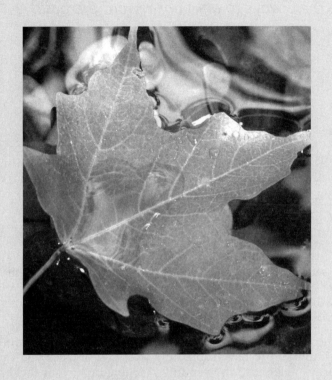

PEDIATRICS

88

Are there ways to affirm or reward the positive behaviors our pediatric patients do in taking care of their diabetes?

 Tip

When gathering information, doing the physical assessment, setting goals, and teaching, we believe it is important to recognize our patients' efforts in taking care of themselves. We offer some examples below:

- "You are doing a nice job of rotating your injection sites. Your skin looks very smooth, and there are no areas of buildup from using one area too much."

- "I see you are wearing your ID bracelet. That is very important in case you needed help for a low blood glucose and were unable to ask for it."

- "Can you show me what you carry to treat a low blood glucose? I am glad to see you carry something with you. It is important to have something with you because you can't always make it to the vending machine or to your locker when your blood glucose is low."

- "Your nails are trimmed nicely to the contour of your toes. They are not too short or too long."

- "Thank you for bringing in your logbook with your numbers. This information tells us how we can work together to make sure your plan is working for you."

We use a variety of small rewards (e.g., stickers, a toy from a treasure chest, a pouch for supplies, T-shirts, gift certificates, movie tickets) to acknowledge the work they do everyday. Sometimes we will write a letter to a high school counselor for a teen's participation in an educational program or a community talk. This can be added to the teen's portfolio of extracurricular activities. We have even documented the hours spent in a diabetes self-management education program and written a letter to a

Tip *Continued*

counselor requesting that community resource credit be given to teens who participate in these programs.

We celebrate our patients' accomplishments by sending a card, clipping a newspaper article, or acknowledging them in our newsletter. We always let our pediatric patients know that we are glad to see them.

89

*H*ow can I help a family that is not involved enough in their child's care and leaves the child with too much responsibility?

 Tip

Some parents aren't involved enough in their child's care because they are overwhelmed by other issues in their lives: other children in the family, their jobs, relationship issues, financial concerns, etc. Sometimes the parent has difficulty learning diabetes management and delegates care to the child or an older sibling. Although many families are often very proud that their young child can "do everything themselves," sometimes these children do not have adequate supervision or support for their diabetes management.

Young children need an adult with them while they are monitoring their blood glucose and taking their insulin. A young child usually does not have the psychomotor or cognitive skills to mix insulins safely. If the insulin is drawn up by the parent or if the child is using an insulin pen, he or she may be able the give the injection by himself or herself. However, an adult must be present during the injection to ensure that the child receives the insulin. An adult also needs to be sure that the child is eating an adequate diet that is consistent in carbohydrates. Make sure that the patient's family understands these responsibilities and knows that you are available to support them.

90

__W__hat can I do about the "overinvolved" parent who will not let his or her child make decisions or participate in his or her care?

 Tip

Parents need to be actively involved in their child's diabetes management. They need to understand the current regimen, including the meal plan, insulin dose, and monitoring. Children also need to participate in their care and assume increasing responsibility each year that they live with diabetes. Some parents are too involved because they are afraid that something will happen to their child if they are not providing the care themselves. They may need help in seeing the value of giving up some control in order to help their child be more independent. As the educator, you can offer guidance in this area for the child and the family. First, you will need to determine what components of diabetes management the parents are doing and what components the child is doing. List these tasks, and then ask the child and parents if some can be shifted. For example, most preschoolers can help with blood glucose monitoring by picking which site to use, helping to get the blood on the strip, and cooperating with the procedure. School-age children can be more actively involved and often take great pride in being "independent." Monitoring blood glucose, giving shots, and counting carbohydrates are skills in which the child six to twelve years of age can become proficient. Most teenagers want to do the care themselves and don't want their parents "running their lives."

If parents are doing all the care for an 8-year-old patient you might respond, "Nathan is 8 years old now, and many children his age are more involved with their care. Nathan, what do you think about doing your own blood glucose monitoring at lunch at school? Mom and Dad, what do you think?"

90

Tip *Continued*

There are other things you can do to support the child's independence. It is important to direct some questions to the child at each encounter with the family. Elicit information from both the child and the parent. Help families understand the need to support their child and share in the care. Doing all of the care for the child gives the child the message that he or she is not capable of doing it and keeps the child in a dependent position. Parents may need help taking a step back to enable their child to take increasing responsibility for his or her care.

91

So many of our families of very young children with diabetes find parenting a young child and taking care of their child's diabetes overwhelming. How can I help?

 Tip

Caring for an infant or toddler is overwhelming enough, and diabetes greatly compounds these feelings. Listen to the family's issues and concerns. Affirm their feelings. Acknowledge how difficult it is to manage diabetes and care for a very young child. Address their specific issues and concerns. The infant's developmental task is learning to trust care providers and his or her environment. There needs to be lots of affection: hugs, kisses, and holding to balance the pain of pokes and shots. Infants generally have a higher target blood glucose range (80–200) to avoid severe low blood glucose.

Developmental classes can be very helpful for these families. Gathering parents with children of similar ages together in a class or clinic is very effective because they can share what is working for them and support each other.

92

*D*o you have specific advice for working with parents who have an infant with diabetes?

 Tip

Specific diabetes management issues to cover when working with parents of an infant include

- the fact that, as parents, they are "on call" 24 hours a day

- how the child may need a three- to four-hour flexible feeding schedule

- a flexible insulin regimen and how it may be helpful

- the challenges involved in managing sporadic and spontaneous physical activity, growth spurts, food intake, and insulin

- a child's inability to recognize and communicate symptoms of hypoglycemia

- ways to treat low blood glucose—gel, cakemate, Karo syrup, juice, or 1/4 cc milk–glucagon

- frequent blood glucose monitoring and how alternate site testing may be helpful

- small doses of insulin and how they may need diluted insulin, e.g., u10 insulin, and 1/3-cc syringes with short needles

- the fact that diabetic ketoacidosis and dehydration can develop rapidly and that infants are more vulnerable to ketones and high blood glucose during acute infections (as evidenced by a fever) such as the flu and ear infections

- how day care providers, babysitters, and extended family members may need to participate in care and be knowledgeable about diabetes

- the fact that support for family members (perhaps through support groups) are vital for successful management

93

***D**o you have specific advice for working with the parent of a toddler?*

 Tip

Toddlers are exploring their environment. They are beginning to walk and move around. Increased activity may cause more erratic blood glucose. They also are beginning to talk. "No!" and "Me!" are two of their favorite words. Power struggles over their blood glucose checks and injections may be common.

Specific diabetes management issues for toddlers include

- gaining a sense of mastery over their environment
- target blood glucose of 80–200
- an erratic appetite
- flexible insulin dosing and how it may be helpful
- oppositional behaviors and power struggles
- the need to create a predictable environment including a specific time and place for blood glucose checks and injections
- ways play therapy can provide an outlet for their feelings, for example, a teddy bear who has diabetes too
- why support from groups, friends, and family is essential

94

Do you have specific advice for working with a family with a preschool-aged child with diabetes?

 Tip

Preschool-aged children are dealing with separation issues and exploring and testing their environment through their play. They are concerned with issues of body integrity. Magical thinking—thinking or wishing something and making it happen—is active during this developmental period. Having a predictable routine is especially helpful for the very young child. The child knows what to expect, and there is security in the predictability of the environment. But children at a very young age can begin to participate in their care. The preschool-aged child may help with blood glucose monitoring by choosing which area to poke, getting the blood on the strip, and watching the numbers come up on the meter.

Diabetes management issues for the preschooler include

- targeting blood glucose at 80–200
- providing a consistent supportive environment
- reassuring them that they did nothing to cause diabetes and that they are not being punished
- providing an outlet for their feelings—play therapy
- accommodating food jags (i.e., periods when children want to eat the same foods again and again)—offer choices
- expecting appetite changes with growth spurts
- giving choices whenever possible to increase a sense of control over their environment (e.g., injection sites, monitoring sites, food)
- providing a predictable environment and routine
- praising them for their cooperation with care—hugs, kisses, stickers, etc.
- offering support—groups, extended family, friends, other families with children of the same age

*D*o you have specific advice for working with
school-aged children with diabetes?

 Tip

The school-aged child is usually fun to work with! They are very
industrious, like rules, are good at technical skills, are beginning to
understand cause and effect relationships, and have increasing independence. The child and parent can learn together. Children at this age can
observe a demonstration of self-care skills and then practice the skills on
a parent and then on themselves. Remember to individualize the teaching, and be sure there is shared responsibility between the parents and the
child.

Diabetes management issues for school-aged children include

- targeting blood glucose at 70–180
- evaluating their physical ability to handle technical self-care
  skills
- beginning the transition to self-care skill based on the
  individual child
- sharing care is the key to success
- providing supervision and guidance
- providing "breaks" from care
- affirming normalcy by treating the child with diabetes like
  other children in the family, including limit-setting
- educating school personnel
- encouraging diabetes camp to provide the opportunity to
  practice self-care skills and interact with other children with
  diabetes

96

How do you know when it's time for diabetes care to transition from the parents to the child?

 Tip

There is no one way because this transition is different for each child and family. Children learn by watching the people in their environment. The transition of responsibility for self-management usually occurs gradually over time. Parents always need some participation in their child's care. The younger the child, the more supervision and direct care is needed. Parental participation can range from providing care for the very young child to helping with problem-solving and integrating self-care skills into an active lifestyle for the adolescent or older teen.

As the child's skills and cognitive abilities increase, the ability to take on more of his or her care increases. From ages six through twelve, children can be taught the skills to give injections, draw up insulin, mix insulin, count carbohydrates, and begin to take on the more complex decision-making of diabetes care. Parents need to be available to supervise, coach, and mentor their child with their new skills. They also need to monitor for signs of stress and be sure that the child does not have too much responsibility for their age.

*D*o you have any specific advice for working
with teenagers with diabetes?

 Tip

Teenagers are striving for independence and autonomy from the family. The peer group becomes very important. Along with increased responsibility for decision-making, this is a time of rapid growth and psychological unrest, which can make blood glucose difficult to manage. Take an interest in the teen as an individual. Learn what he or she likes to do so you can tailor diabetes care to fit his or her lifestyle. Provide teaching and support for both the teen and the parents.

Diabetes management issues for adolescents include

- targeting blood glucose at 70–150

- providing options for management

- discussing how increased flexibility in treatment (e.g., through an insulin pump or multiple daily injection therapy) requires increased decision-making and monitoring

- discussing safety issues with regard to diabetes (e.g., driving, alcohol, and contraception/sexual activity)

- providing options for medical ID

- offering support at each encounter

- focusing education on decision-making and coping skills

- providing care and classes in a developmentally staged paradigm (i.e., classes for teens separate from parents)

- offering a class for parents that is separate from teens but that discusses the same topics (i.e., parallel peer support group format)

98

Many of our older teens are ready to move to adult care providers. How can I help them make a smooth transition?

 Tip

Transitioning care from the pediatric to the adult health care system requires some preparation. As adolescents prepare for college or life after high school, the health care team needs to help them plan how their care will be managed. Different providers handle this differently. In some practices/institutions, there is a young adult clinic staffed by both adult and pediatric team members to ease this transition of care. Where resources do not allow for this arrangement, some patients are transitioned to adult providers when they turn 18, whereas in other settings, care is given by their pediatric providers until they graduate from college. The team and the patient need to decide what will work best for each patient. This is very individual, and there is not one "right" way. Making sure that the patient is well cared for is what is important.

Helping people at this age become "adult" consumers of health care is critical. They are probably used to their parents fulfilling this role. Teach young adults and older teens what the standards of care are for the person with diabetes: frequency of office visits, expectations for office visits, frequency of lab work, appropriate screening tests, and the importance of ongoing education. Stress the importance of their role as a collaborator in their care and their responsibility for ensuring that standards are met. Encourage participation in a diabetes self-management education program as an update or a refresher course when transitioning to an adult provider. Provide sources of information (e.g., *Diabetes Forecast* and www.diabetes.org) to stay abreast of diabetes care and new developments.

*W*hat is the best way to help children manage
their diabetes when they are at school?

 Tip

Helping parents to build a partnership with the school is a good place to start. Some school personnel are intimidated or afraid of having a child with diabetes in their care. Providing appropriate materials and education for school personnel helps to smooth the way. Encourage parents to meet with teachers and other school personnel each year before school starts and explain what is necessary for their child during the school day. Situations that classroom teachers need to be able to handle include

- school parties—extra food and treats
- field trips and outings—scheduling issues
- exercise, gym, and recess—covering with extra carbohydrates
- monitoring—who, what, when, where, how, and why
- treating mild low blood glucose—how this child might act and how to respond
- importance of treating the child with diabetes as all other children in the classroom are treated

100

How can I help a family when the school is unwilling to accommodate the needs of the child with diabetes?

 Tip

Federal law protects children with special needs, including those with diabetes, to assure them a "free appropriate education." A formalized plan called a "504" plan (Section 504 of the Rehabilitation Act of 1973) can be written up to outline the accommodations that the child requires in school. This "504" should include all pertinent information for this individual child in this particular school. The diabetes care plan should include

- where supplies will be kept (blood glucose monitoring, ketone testing, insulin, snacks)
- where blood glucose monitoring will be done
- who will supervise monitoring, insulin administration, etc.
- where insulin will be administered if needed
- symptoms of low blood glucose and how to treat
- symptoms of high blood glucose and how to treat
- timing of meals and snacks
- how to handle emergencies

The ADA web site, www.diabetes.org, has resources for working with schools. One patient education brochure is *Your School & Your Rights*, which outlines the rights of children with diabetes in schools. Many states are working on legislation or other programs to help schools better understand and accommodate children with diabetes.

101

Many of our pediatric patients with diabetes have divorced parents and spend half of their time with one set of parents and the other half of their time with the other set of parents. How can I be sure the child gets adequate care with both families?

 Tip

Sometimes these situations create stress and confusion, and the diabetes can get lost in the shuffle. The educator's role can be to focus on fostering open communication between the families around the diabetes management. It is important that all adults responsible for the child with diabetes have a thorough understanding of diabetes and that child's management plan.

- Have both sets of parents attend and complete a diabetes self-management education program specific to the needs of the pediatric patient and their families (especially the "cooks")

- Give prescriptions to cover adequate supplies for both homes (insulin, syringes, monitoring supplies, ketone test trips, glucagon emergency kits, etc.)

- Create a management plan and goals with the child and both families that they can agree on and that will work for them

- Write down the instructions and the plan and give a copy to the child and both families

- Encourage a parent from each family to attend office visits with the child

- Make sure that the school or day care has the pertinent information and contact numbers for families in case of emergencies

I Bonus

Support is such an important part of living with diabetes. How can I help parents and children get the support they need?

 Tip

"Support is in the eye of the beholder." Individuals seek the kind of support that gives them comfort. The definition of support is different for each person. Helping each patient find out what works is the key. The following questions are designed to assess what support is needed: information, education, social support, a care provider, etc. Finding answers to these questions may help patients and families identify their existing or potential support.

- Who are supportive individuals in your environment? Can you ask them for help?

- Do you belong to a church or other community group?

- Is your nuclear family supportive? Is your extended family supportive and available?

- Do you belong to a diabetes support group?

- Are there friends who can listen and help?

- Is there an on-going diabetes education program available to you?

- Is your diabetes treatment team supportive and helpful?

- Are parents of children with diabetes able to get away for some time alone together?

- Are there other families with a child who has diabetes who can be supportive and swap babysitting for evenings out?

- Is diabetes camp available for children and families?

About the Authors

Robert M. Anderson, EdD, is an educational psychologist with 22 years of experience in diabetes research and education. He is an NIH-funded research scientist with the Michigan Diabetes Research and Training Center and professor of medical education at the University of Michigan Medical School. He has won a number of honors and awards for his work in diabetes education.

Martha Mitchell Funnell, MS, RN, CDE, is a clinical nurse specialist and diabetes educator at the University of Michigan Diabetes Research and Training Center. She has won a number of honors and awards for her work in the areas of patient empowerment, patient education, and curriculum development. She is the American Diabetes Association's 2002–2003 President, Health Care & Education.

Nugget T. Burkhart, RN, MA, CPNP, CDE, is a practitioner in the Department of Pediatric Endocrinology at the University of Michigan. She coordinates the University of Michigan "Pump Team," a program for children and adolescents on insulin pump therapy. She works closely with children and their families to tailor their diabetes regimen to their specific and ever-changing needs.

Mary Lou Gillard, MS, RN, CDE, is a community nurse educator in the Department of Medical Education at the University of Michigan. She provides Diabetes Self-Management Education in a research setting and is the nurse case manager to those who participate in her program. She has had diabetes for 35 years.

Robin B. Nwankwo, MPH, RD, CDE, is a community dietitian employed by the Department of Medical Education at the University of Michigan. She coordinates grant-funded community complications screening and education programs.

About the American Diabetes Association

The American Diabetes Association is the nation's leading voluntary health organization supporting diabetes research, information, and advocacy. Its mission is to prevent and cure diabetes and to improve the lives of all people affected by diabetes. The American Diabetes Association is the leading publisher of comprehensive diabetes information. Its huge library of practical and authoritative books for people with diabetes covers every aspect of self-care—cooking and nutrition, fitness, weight control, medications, complications, emotional issues, and general self-care.

To order American Diabetes Association books: Call 1-800-232-6733. http://store.diabetes.org [Note: there is no need to use **www** when typing this particular Web address]

To join the American Diabetes Association: Call 1-800-806-7801. www.diabetes.org/membership

For more information about diabetes or ADA programs and services: Call 1-800-342-2383. E-mail: Customerservice@diabetes.org www.diabetes.org

To locate an ADA/NCQA Recognized Provider of quality diabetes care in your area: www.ncqa.org/dprp

To find an ADA Recognized Education Program in your area: Call 1-888-232-0822. www.diabetes.org/recognition/education.asp

To join the fight to increase funding for diabetes research, end discrimination, and improve insurance coverage: Call 1-800-342-2383. www.diabetes.org/advocacy

To find out how you can get involved with the programs in your community: Call 1-800-342-2383. See below for program Web addresses.

- *American Diabetes Month:* Educational activities aimed at those diagnosed with diabetes—month of November. www.diabetes.org/ADM
- *American Diabetes Alert:* Annual public awareness campaign to find the undiagnosed—held the fourth Tuesday in March. www.diabetes.org/alert
- *The Diabetes Assistance & Resources Program (DAR):* diabetes awareness program targeted to the Latino community. www.diabetes.org/ DAR
- *African American Program:* diabetes awareness program targeted to the African American community. www.diabetes.org/africanamerican
- *Awakening the Spirit: Pathways to Diabetes Prevention & Control:* diabetes awareness program targeted to the Native American community. www.diabetes.org/awakening

To find out about an important research project regarding type 2 diabetes: www.diabetes.org/ada/research.asp

To obtain information on making a planned gift or charitable bequest: Call 1-888-700-7029. www.diabetes.org/ada/plan.asp

To make a donation or memorial contribution: Call 1-800-342-2383. www.diabetes.org/ada/cont.asp